ADDRESSING THE NATION'S CHANGING NEEDS FOR BIOMEDICAL AND BEHAVIORAL SCIENTISTS

Committee on National Needs
for Biomedical and Behavioral Scientists

Education and Career Studies Unit

Office of Scientific and Engineering Personnel

National Research Council

NATIONAL ACADEMY PRESS
Washington, DC

NATIONAL ACADEMY PRESS • 2101 Constitution Avenue, N.W. • Washington, DC 20418

NOTICE: The project that is the subject of this report was approved by the Governing Board of the National Research Council, whose members are drawn from the councils of the National Academy of Sciences, the National Academy of Engineering, and the Institute of Medicine. The members of the committee responsible for the report were chosen for their special competences and with regard for appropriate balance.

This study was performed under Contract No. N01-OD-7-2109 between the National Academy of Sciences and the National Institutes of Health. Any opinions, findings, conclusions, or recommendations expressed in this publication are those of the Committee on National Needs for Biomedical and Behavioral Scientists and do not necessarily reflect the view of the agency that provided support for this project.

Additional copies of this report are available from the National Academy Press, 2101 Constitution Avenue, N.W., Box 285, Washington, DC 20055; (800) 624-6242 or (202) 334-3313 (in the Washington metropolitan area); http://www.nap.edu.

Library of Congress Catalog Card Number 00-105076

International Standard Book Number 0-309-06981-5

Printed in the United States of America

THE NATIONAL ACADEMIES

National Academy of Sciences
National Academy of Engineering
Institute of Medicine
National Research Council

The **National Academy of Sciences** is a private, nonprofit, self-perpetuating society of distinguished scholars engaged in scientific and engineering research, dedicated to the furtherance of science and technology and to their use for the general welfare. Upon the authority of the charter granted to it by the Congress in 1863, the Academy has a mandate that requires it to advise the federal government on scientific and technical matters. Dr. Bruce M. Alberts is president of the National Academy of Sciences.

The **National Academy of Engineering** was established in 1964, under the charter of the National Academy of Sciences, as a parallel organization of outstanding engineers. It is autonomous in its administration and in the selection of its members, sharing with the National Academy of Sciences the responsibility for advising the federal government. The National Academy of Engineering also sponsors engineering programs aimed at meeting national needs, encourages education and research, and recognizes the superior achievements of engineers. Dr. William A. Wulf is president of the National Academy of Engineering.

The **Institute of Medicine** was established in 1970 by the National Academy of Sciences to secure the services of eminent members of appropriate professions in the examination of policy matters pertaining to the health of the public. The Institute acts under the responsibility given to the National Academy of Sciences by its congressional charter to be an adviser to the federal government and, upon its own initiative, to identify issues of medical care, research, and education. Dr. Kenneth I. Shine is president of the Institute of Medicine.

The **National Research Council** was organized by the National Academy of Sciences in 1916 to associate the broad community of science and technology with the Academy's purposes of furthering knowledge and advising the federal government. Functioning in accordance with general policies determined by the Academy, the Council has become the principal operating agency of both the National Academy of Sciences and the National Academy of Engineering in providing services to the government, the public, and the scientific and engineering communities. The Council is administered jointly by both Academies and the Institute of Medicine. Dr. Bruce M. Alberts and Dr. William A. Wulf are chairman and vice chairman, respectively, of the National Research Council.

Committee on National Needs for Biomedical and Behavioral Scientists

Howard Hiatt, ***Chair***
Professor of Medicine
Harvard Medical School
Senior Physician
Department of General Medicine
Brigham and Women's Hospital

Gail H. Cassell
Vice President of Infectious Diseases
Eli Lilly and Company

Janice G. Douglas
Professor of Medicine and Physiology and Biophysics
Vice Chair, Academic Affairs
Case Western Reserve University School of Medicine

Richard B. Freeman
Ascherman Professor of Economics
Harvard University

Lee Goldman
Julius R. Krevans Distinguished Professor and Chair
Department of Medicine
Associate Dean for Clinical Affairs
University of California, San Francisco School of Medicine

Leland H. Hartwell
President and Director
Fred Hutchinson Cancer Research Center

John F. Kihlstrom
Professor of Psychology
University of California, Berkeley

Ellen M. Markman
Associate Dean of Social Sciences
Stanford University

Edward E. Penhoet
Dean
School of Public Health
University of California, Berkeley

Steven A. Schroeder
President
Robert Wood Johnson Foundation

Michael S. Teitelbaum
Program Director
Alfred P. Sloan Foundation

Staff
Rodolfo A. Bulatao, Demographer
Charlotte Kuh
Julie Parker, Senior Project Assistant
Jennifer Sutton, Study Director
James A. Voytuk

Office of Scientific and Engineering Personnel Advisory Committee

M. R. C. Greenwood, ***Chair***
Chancellor
University of California, Santa Cruz

John D. Wiley, ***Vice Chair***
Provost and Vice Chancellor for Academic Affairs
University of Wisconsin, Madison

Carlos Gutierrez
Professor of Chemistry
California State University, Los Angeles

Stephen J. Lukasik
Independent Consultant

Ronald G. Ehrenberg
Irving M. Ives Professor of Industrial and Labor Relations and Economics
Cornell University

Edward Penhoet
Dean
School of Public Health
University of California, Berkeley

Tadataka Yamada
Chairman, Research and Development
SmithKline Beecham Pharmaceuticals

A. Thomas Young
Former President and Chief Operating Officer
Martin Marietta Corporation

William H. Miller, ***ex officio***
Department of Chemistry
University of California, Berkeley

Claudia I. Mitchell-Kernan
Vice Chancellor of Academic Affairs and Dean
University of California, Los Angeles

Staff
Charlotte Kuh, Executive Director
Marilyn J. Baker, Associate Executive Director

Preface

This congressionally mandated report on the training of biomedical and behavioral researchers reviews the recent production and current supply of scientists and is the eleventh in a series that began in 1975. It makes recommendations for the size and scope of the National Research Service Award (NRSA) training program in the years ahead. Unlike earlier studies, it also considers research training mechanisms other than NRSA training grants and fellowships. As a result, this report devotes a great deal of attention to the balance between NRSA and non-NRSA training activities and the coordination between the two.

In addition, the report stresses the need for research training programs to keep pace with changes in the organization of science and the economic and social realities of health care. In contrast to the technical and methodological advances in biomedical and behavioral research that are routinely incorporated into research training programs, changes in the organization of science, the delivery of health care, and the nation's demography pose more difficult challenges. Addressing these challenges, which have a bearing on research training overall, will require the active involvement of the National Institutes of Health, the Agency for Healthcare Research and Quality, and the Health Resources and Services Administration to collectively take a more active role in research training.

In particular, the agencies responsible for research training must seek more effective ways to draw greater numbers of physicians and other health care professionals into research careers, to attract and prepare future investigators to address disparities in health status, and to ensure that more investigators in all fields are prepared to conduct interdisciplinary health research.

The report was crafted by a committee of eleven, drawn from the fields of biomedical, behavioral, and clinical research, labor economics, and demography and for the most part represents the consensus of their views. One of our members, however, has offered a personal statement on funding for research and research training in the behavioral and social sciences; his views can be found in Appendix F.

The report also reflects the contributions of numerous others who generously shared their time and expertise. More than a hundred contributors responded to the committee's invitation to submit written comments on research training in the health sciences; their responses are summarized in Appendix C. Many others met with the committee or its chair to provide information and offer suggestions. Among the latter were Norman Anderson, Andrea Baruchin, Carol Bazell, David Blumenthal, Marvin Cassman, John Eisenberg, Suzanne Feetham, Susan Gerbi, Patricia Grady, Steven Hyman, Alan Kraut, Al Lazen, Richard McIntosh, David Nathan, John Norvell, Georgine Pion, Howard Schachman, Harold Slavkin, and Ellen Stover.

The committee is especially grateful to six scientists in training who candidly shared their experiences, including their struggles, in becoming independent investigators: Regis Krah, Krishna Mallik, John Otridge, Julie Ann Sosa, James Rowlett, and Marc Weisskopf. We wish them great success in their careers.

This report was made possible by funding from the National Institutes of Health and the willingness of scores of staff members throughout the National Institutes of Health, the Agency for Healthcare Research and Quality, and the Health Resources and Services Administration to provide valuable information. At the National Institutes of Health, we are particularly indebted to Walter Schaffer, the project officer, for his patient guidance and good counsel, Deputy Director Ruth Kirschstein for her generosity with her thoughts and her time, and Robert Moore and Carol Bleakley of the Office of Reports and Analysis for the graciousness with which they fulfilled our repeated requests for data.

The committee owes special thanks to Don McMaster and his colleagues at Quantum Research Corporation for their skillful data analyses and to the staff members of many professional associations and societies who readily and generously shared their extensive knowledge. Among the groups providing information to the committee were the American Association of Colleges of Nursing, the American Dental Association, the American Medical Association, the American Psychological Association, the American Psychological Society, the Association for Health Services Research, the Association of American Medical Colleges, the Association of American Dental Schools, the Association of American Universities, the American Society for Cell Biology, the Council of Graduate Schools, and the Federation of American Societies for Experimental Biology.

Much information in this report is drawn from national surveys of doctoral scientists conducted under the direction of the National Science Foundation, with funding from a number of federal agencies, including the National Institutes of Health. The use of these data, of course, does not imply National Science Foundation endorsement of our research methods or conclusions.

This report has been reviewed in draft form by individuals chosen for their diverse perspectives and technical expertise, in accordance with procedures approved by the NRC's Report Review Committee. The purpose of this independent review is to provide candid and critical comments that will assist the institution in making the published report as sound as possible and to ensure that the report meets institutional standards for objectivity, evidence, and responsiveness to the study charge. The review comments and draft manuscript remain confidential to protect the integrity of the deliberative process. We wish to thank the following individuals for their participation in the review of this report: Ralph M. Garruto, State University of New York at Binghamton; Ira Herskowitz, University of California, San Francisco; Lyle V. Jones, University of North Carolina, Chapel Hill; William J. Koopman, University of Alabama at Birmingham; Georgine M. Pion, Vanderbilt University; Samuel H. Preston, University of Pennsylvania; Shirley M. Tilghman, Princeton University; Jean D. Wilson, University of Texas Southwestern Medical Center; and Tadataka Yamada, SmithKline Beecham Corporation. While these reviewers provided constructive comments and suggestions, it must be emphasized that responsibility for the final content of this report rests entirely with the authoring committee and the institution.

The National Research Council staff members who contributed to this study are too numerous to acknowledged in a brief preface. We are especially indebted to Rodolfo Bulatao for the tirelessness and good grace with which he carried out the demographic analyses and drafted Appendix D of this report. James Voytuk ably generated volumes of data on behalf of the committee and patiently lent his expertise to their interpretation. Julie Parker, Edvin Hernandez, Peggy Petrochenkov, and Shirel Smith all cheerfully dedicated long hours to the preparation and production of this report.

Finally, a few words about Jennifer Sutton, the study director. The committee knows well (and I far more) that this report is in very large part attributable to her competence, thoughtfulness, seemingly inexhaustible energy, good humor, and tireless and effective management of the obstacles that arose, and warm and generous relations with the many on whom we called.

Howard Hiatt
Chair

Contents

FIGURES, TABLES, AND BOXES

Figures

Tables

Box

Executive Summary

This report, the eleventh in a series on national needs for biomedical and behavioral research scientists, appears at a time of contradictions. On the one hand, improvements in health resulting from biomedical and behavioral research are increasingly apparent: the sharp decline in the death rate from AIDS, great improvements in survival rates from heart disease, and more effective treatments for cancer, among others. Advances in the understanding of many diseases, including those of the nervous system, promise rapid progress in prevention and management.

On the other hand, it is increasingly difficult for new scientists to establish independent research careers. Every year there is considerable disparity between the number of new Ph.D.s, particularly in the basic biomedical sciences, and available positions for faculty and other research professionals. The need is growing for clinical scientists who can help translate research findings into improvements in health. Yet the economic barriers to establishing a clinical research career are formidable, and clinical research itself is increasingly difficult to carry out as medical care becomes progressively more cost conscious.

Moreover, the composition of the research workforce and the focus of its work do not adequately address some of the nation's needs. For example, although medically underserved minority populations are rapidly increasing, the number of research personnel who seek to address their health problems is not growing commensurately.

CHARGE TO THE COMMITTEE

Against this background, the National Institutes of Health (NIH) asked the Committee on National Needs for Biomedical and Behavioral Scientists to assess the need for National Research Service Award training grants and fellowships and the need for new research personnel in the biomedical, behavioral, and clinical sciences. Specifically, the committee was charged with:

- estimating the current and future supply of scientists;
- estimating the future demand for scientists;
- utilizing estimates of the future demand for scientists and information about the current balance between supply and demand to develop recommendations for the appropriate size of the NRSA program and the overall production of research personnel; and
- developing recommendations for improving the NRSA program.

FINDINGS AND RECOMMENDATIONS

The committee concentrated on the three broad fields of biomedical, behavioral, and clinical research, with dental, nursing, and health services research included in the latter category. A number of the committee's recommendations were based on the results of a demographic analysis of the research workforce. This analysis considered such factors as the average age of current investigators in the biomedical and behavioral sciences, the number of Ph.D.s expected to join the workforce in the years ahead, and the likely effect of retirements and deaths. The committee also reviewed such indicators of short-term demand as trends in faculty and industry hiring and perceptions of the job market by recent Ph.D.s.

As described in Chapter 2, the committee found that the number of new Ph.D.s awarded annually in the basic biomedical sciences is well above that needed to keep pace with growth in the U.S. economy and to replace those leaving the workforce as a result of retirement and death. Moreover, many recent entrants to the biomedical workforce are working in postdoctoral or other temporary positions. **From its review of these and other trends in the education and employment of basic biomedical scientists, the committee concluded that research training and overall Ph.D. production in these fields should not be increased.**

In its assessment of the behavioral and social science workforce in Chapter 3, the committee found that the number of new Ph.D.s awarded annually in these fields is also sufficient to keep pace with growth in the U.S. economy and to replace those leaving the workforce as a result of retirement and death. Job prospects for new Ph.D.s in the behavioral and social sciences have improved since the early 1990s, but faculty hiring is still below the levels of the late 1980s. The extent to which these findings apply to the portion of the behavioral and social science workforce that focuses on health research is less clear, but the committee found no reason to believe that circumstances differ for this group of investigators. **As a result of its review of trends in the education and employment of behavioral and social scientists, the committee also concluded that research training and overall Ph.D. production in these fields should not be increased.**

In its examination of the clinical research workforce, described in Chapter 4, the committee found two disparate trends. Since 1975, Ph.D.s awarded in clinical science fields have increased at a rate faster than in the biomedical or behavioral sciences. Though data on M.D.s, dentists, and other health care doctorates in clinical research available to the committee were much more limited than on Ph.D.s, there was clear evidence of a decline in the number of M.D.s conducting research. The mounting indebtedness of medical students and other economic disincentives are likely contributing factors. **Its review of trends in the composition of the clinical research workforce led the committee to recommend that Ph.D. production in the clinical science fields not be increased but that efforts to train and retain physicians be intensified until the decline in the numbers has been reversed and the clinical research workforce includes substantially more M.D.s than is now the case.**

As discussed in Chapters 2 and 3, the committee concluded that while the number of Ph.D.s produced annually in the biomedical and behavioral sciences should not increase, enormous opportunities exist for more broadly trained investigators. Unlike research grants, where the focus is appropriately on the quality of research, NRSA programs permit attention to and monitoring of the breadth and quality of the training that students and fellows receive. **Because of the successful career outcomes of NRSA participants and the program's tradition of multidisciplinary training, the committee recommended that the NIH gradually expand its funding of NRSA training grants and fellowships and proportionately reduce its funding of graduate research assistantships.**

As noted throughout the report and addressed in more detail in Chapter 5, the committee found African Americans, Hispanics, and Native Americans to be greatly underrepresented among Ph.D.s and health professionals in the research workforce. Meanwhile, the health problems of the nation's growing underrepresented minority populations are not receiving adequate attention. Addressing these problems will require both more minority scientists in biomedical and behavioral research and more minority and nonminority investigators turning their attention to disparities in health. **To ensure that the composition of the research workforce and the focus of its work address the nation's needs, the committee urges the NIH, the Agency for Healthcare Quality and Research, and the Health Resources and Services Administration to more carefully examine the results of existing policies and programs intended to increase the diversity of the research workforce. Only those that are effective merit continuation or increase. Further, the committee recommends that the agencies support activities to improve opportunities for minority students in secondary schools, an educational level outside the scope of the existing NRSA program.**

As discussed in Chapter 5, the committee recognizes that achieving these goals will require the NIH, the Agency for Healthcare Quality and Research, and the Health Resources and Services Administration to consolidate and increase their oversight of research training and training-related activities. **The committee believes that enhanced oversight of research training will lead to the preparation of a workforce that better reflects the nation's needs and more scientists who are prepared for the increasingly interdisciplinary nature of research.**

The committee appreciates the profound benefits that have accrued to the nation as a result of NRSA training programs. Although NRSA funding now accounts for the training of a much smaller share of the nation's biomedical, clinical, and behavioral science workforce than when the program began, the NIH, the Agency for Healthcare Quality and Research, and the Health Resources and Services Administration continue to have a great influence on the quality and quantity of health research personnel trained in the U.S. The committee believes that the steps summarized above, and described in more detail in Chapters 2 through 5, will help these agencies to broaden their training activities and thereby address more comprehensively the health problems of today and tomorrow.

1

Introduction

Since the National Research Council released its last evaluation of workforce needs in the biomedical and behavioral sciences in 1994, the continuing contributions of researchers to the nation's health have touched the lives of millions of Americans. A striking example was the sharp decline in the death rate from AIDS in 1997, a result of more than a decade of research on the disease and on strategies for its prevention and treatment. Mortality from AIDS now stands at the lowest level in the United States since data were first collected in 1987.[1]

With the designation of the 1990s as the Decade of the Brain,[2] researchers have focused attention on disorders of the brain, such as autism, schizophrenia, and impairments in speech, language, and hearing. At the same time, advances in imaging techniques have provided investigators with noninvasive approaches for observing the living brain, allowing them to study normal functioning as well as damage and disorder. Notable advances over the last half of the 1990s included the identification of genes associated with the development of degenerative disorders such as Alzheimer's, Parkinson's, and Huntington's diseases; new medications for depression, anxiety, and bipolar disorder; and the increasing use of more effective treatments to lessen the damage of spinal injuries and stroke.[3]

Of great significance as well are the improvements in health that were celebrated when two of the National Institutes of Health's (NIH) oldest institutes marked their fiftieth anniversaries: the National Heart, Lung, and Blood Institute and the National Institute of Dental and Craniofacial Research. Since they were established as the second and third institutes in 1948, research has transformed the practice of both medicine and dentistry.

If a heart attack did not result in early death 50 years ago—as it did for one-third of patients who reached the hospital—it often marked the end of an active life. In the late 1940s, treatment for a heart attack was often limited to pain control and bed rest. Many patients were not permitted to sit up in a chair for many weeks.[4] At the time, heart disease and its associated conditions were by far the largest single cause for retirement under the disability provisions of the Civil Service Retirement Act.[5]

The age-adjusted rate of death from coronary heart disease has decreased by more than half over the past 30 years as a result of increased public awareness and adoption of lifestyles that reduce heart disease (especially decreased tobacco use), medications that control

[1] Ventura, Stephanie J., Robert N. Anderson, Joyce A. Martin, and Betty L. Smith. *Births and Deaths: Preliminary Data for 1997.* National Vital Statistics Reports 47, no. 4. Hyattsville, Md.: National Center for Health Statistics, 1998.

[2] President George Bush. Proclamation. "Decade of the Brain, 1990-1999, Proclamation 6158." *Federal Register* 55, no. 140 (1990): 29553.

[3] Dana Alliance for Brain Initiatives. *Update 1998: Reshaping Expectations.* New York: Dana Press, 1998.

[4] National Institutes of Health. National Heart, Lung, and Blood Institute. *Scientific Advances: Heart Attack and Counterattack.* Bethesda, Md.: NIH, 1998.

[5] Lenfant, Claude. "Heart Research: Celebration and Renewal." *Circulation* 96, no. 11 (1997): 3822–23.

high blood pressure and cholesterol, and such advances in diagnostics, treatment, and surgery as stress tests, "clotbuster" drugs, and balloon angioplasty.[6] Improvements in treatment now allow most survivors to return to normal activities within weeks of a heart attack.

Similarly, the anniversary of the National Institute of Dental and Craniofacial Research provided an opportunity to reflect on the enormous improvements in oral health over the last half century. At the outbreak of World War II, almost 10 percent of military-age American men were ineligible for the draft because they had less than six opposing teeth in each jaw.[7] Most people living in the U.S. at the time could expect to be toothless by the age of 45.[8] Today, the combination of fluoridated drinking water, dental sealants, and other improvements in prevention and treatment allow the majority of Americans to retain their teeth throughout their lives.

Beyond the latest improvements in medical care and health brought about by their research, investigators are also contributing to the nation's economy in new ways. The rise of cost-effectiveness studies (which may eventually help guide health care spending)[9,10] is one example; another, much further advanced, is evident in the field of biotechnology. After a period of steep growth—and occasional setbacks—in the 1980s, the biotechnology industry is now on firm footing and turning out new products at a rapid pace. Of the 65 drugs developed by biotechnology companies on the market in 1998, half had been introduced in the previous two years and the Food and Drug Administration is reviewing another 200.[11]

ORIGINS OF THE NATIONAL RESEARCH SERVICE AWARD PROGRAM

Many roots of today's research training programs in the biomedical and behavioral sciences extend back to 1930 and the beginnings of the NIH. The enactment of the Ransdell Act that year established the NIH as the focus of the growing research activities of the Public Health Service and assigned the new agency a role in maintaining the research workforce. Recognizing that the agency would require a supply of trained personnel to fulfill its mission, legislators provided for the NIH to award fellowships to investigators interested in conducting research.[12]

Before the decade was out, the first of NIH's "categorical" institutes had been founded, and the agency's duties had been expanded to include advanced clinical training as well. In establishing the National Cancer Institute in 1937, Congress charged it with providing "training and instruction in technical matters relating to the diagnosis and treatment of cancer,"[13] along with research training. As additional institutes were formed (the National Heart Institute and the National Institute for Dental Research in 1948, the National Institute of Mental Health in 1949, and the National Institute of Arthritis and Metabolic Diseases and the National Institute of Neurological Diseases and Blindness in 1950), their training responsibilities were based to a large degree on those established for the National Cancer Institute.[14] As a result, for much of its first two decades, NIH training support was divided between clinical and research training.

By the mid-1950s, NIH policymakers concluded that medical specialty training in most fields could be sustained without continuing NIH support, and the agency

[6] National Institutes of Health. National Heart, Lung, and Blood Institute. *Scientific Advances: Heart Attack and Counterattack.* Bethesda, Md.: NIH, 1998.

[7] Harris, Ruth Roy. *Dental Science in a New Age: A History of the National Institute of Dental Research.* Rockville, Md.: Montrose Press, 1989.

[8] U.S. Congress. House. Committee on Appropriations. Subcommittee on Labor, Health and Human Services, and Education. *Statement by Dr. Harold Slavkin on Fiscal Year 1999 President's Budget Request for the National Institute of Dental Research.* 17 March 1998.

[9] Berman, Stephen, Patricia J. Byrns, Jessica Bondy, Pamela J. Smith, and Dennis Lezotte. "Otitis Media-Related Antibiotic Prescribing Patterns, Outcomes, and Expenditures in a Pediatric Medicaid Population." *Pediatrics* 100, no. 4 (1997): 585-92.

[10] Gleason, Patrick P., Wishwa N. Kapoor, Roslyn A. Stone, Judith R. Lave, D. Scott Obrosky, Richard Schulz, Daniel E. Singer, Christopher M. Coley, Thomas J. Marrie, and Michael J. Fine. "Medical Outcomes and Antimicrobial Costs with the Use of the American Thoracic Society Guidelines for Outpatients with Community-Acquired Pneumonia." *JAMA* 278, no. 1 (1997): 32-39.

[11] McDonald, Duff, Pablo Galarza, and Sarah Rose. "The Biotech Boom." *Money* (September 1998): 83-98.

[12] National Institutes of Health. Task Forces for the Review of NIH Biomedical Research. *Review of the National Institutes of Health Biomedical Research Training Programs.* Bethesda, Md.: NIH, 1989.

[13] Ibid.

[14] U.S. Congress. Senate. Committee on Labor and Public Welfare. *National Research Service Award Act of 1974.* 93rd Cong., 1st sess., 1973. S. Rept. 93-381.

returned to its earlier emphasis on research training.[15] This change was followed by the formation of the Division of General Medical Sciences in 1958 and by a redistribution of research training responsibilities among the NIH institutes. As the new division (later an institute itself) took over responsibility for predoctoral training in the basic biomedical sciences, the categorical institutes increasingly focused on postdoctoral research training for Ph.D.s and physicians in the areas most closely allied with their missions. The only exception was the National Institute of Mental Health, which continued to support predoctoral training in the behavioral sciences.[16]

By 1968 about 15 percent of NIH extramural research funding was dedicated to research training programs, and the agency was supporting the training of some 16,000 new investigators each year. But by this time, growing inflation and the Vietnam war were taking a toll on the federal budget, and spending for domestic programs, including research and research training, was subjected to heightened scrutiny.[17,18] After several years of fiscal constraint, the federal budget proposed by President Nixon in 1973 eliminated funding for the NIH's training grant and fellowship awards. The NIH was not the only target; the National Science Foundation's research training grants had already been slated to be phased out as well.[19]

In making the case for eliminating the NIH's training programs, the Nixon administration cited several significant concerns. With the NIH receiving many more applications for research grants than it had funds to support, administration officials contended that the supply of investigators was more than sufficient to carry out the agency's research mission and that the NIH's responsibilities for building up the research workforce had been fulfilled. Furthermore, many of those undergoing research training did not pursue careers in either academics or research but instead established private practices as medical specialists or clinical psychologists.[20] Though not explicitly stated, some believed that the Nixon administration's greatest concern was that training new investigators at the same pace as in the past would create a continuing cycle of pressure for increases in research funding.[21]

For their part, universities, faculty, and their professional organizations vigorously objected to the White House proposal, maintaining that their concerns did not merit such drastic measures. Ultimately, Congress entered the debate, holding hearings and initiating legislative action. The result was the National Research Service Award Act of 1974,[22] which consolidated the research training activities then sponsored by the NIH and the Alcohol, Drug Abuse, and Mental Health Administration into a single inclusive program of training grants and fellowships: the National Research Service Awards. The National Science Foundation, however, did not fare so well; its program of research training grants was eliminated in 1973.[23]

Yet supportive as it was of the NIH and its sister agency, the Alcohol, Drug Abuse, and Mental Health Administration (ADAMHA), Congress shared some of the Nixon administration's reservations about the management of research training support.[24] As a result, legislators incorporated measures into the National Research Service Award Act to ensure that the new training program would be equitably administered and responsive to the needs of research. From the outset, Congress signaled its intent that the National Research Service Award (NRSA) program should treat its participants evenhandedly and eliminate the "discrepancy in stipends paid to Ph.D. as opposed to M.D. graduate students"[25] that existed in the earlier NIH training pro-

---

[15] Shannon, James A. *Federal Support of Biomedical Sciences: Development and Academic Impact.* Washington, D.C.: Association of American Medical Colleges, 1976.

[16] U.S. Congress. Senate. Committee on Labor and Public Welfare. *National Research Service Award Act of 1974.* 93rd Cong., 1st sess., 1973. S. Rept. 93-381.

[17] Strickland, Stephen Parks. *Research and the Health of Americans.* Boston: D. C. Heath and Company, 1978.

[18] Shannon, James A. *Federal Support of Biomedical Sciences: Development and Academic Impact.* Washington, D.C.: Association of American Medical Colleges, 1976.

[19] Walsh, John. "NIH Training Grants: The Uncertainty Factor." *Science* 188, no. 4193 (1975): 1092-94.

[20] Strickland, Stephen Parks. *Research and the Health of Americans.* Boston: D. C. Heath, 1978.

[21] Shannon, James A. *Federal Support of Biomedical Sciences: Development and Academic Impact.* Washington, D.C.: Association of American Medical Colleges, 1976.

[22] U.S. Congress. Senate. Committee on Labor and Public Welfare. *National Research Service Award Act of 1974.* 93rd Cong., 1st sess., 1973. S. Rept. 93-381.

[23] National Science Foundation. *Twenty-second Annual Report for Fiscal Year 1972.* Washington, D.C.: NSF, 1973.

[24] Walsh, John. "NIH Training Grants: The Uncertainty Factor." *Science* 188, no. 4193 (1975): 1092-94.

[25] U.S. Congress. Senate. Committee on Labor and Public Welfare. *National Research Service Award Act of 1974.* 93rd Cong., 1st sess., 1973. S. Rept. 93-381.

grams. Legislators also took steps to discourage individuals from going into medical specialties or other nonresearch careers following their training by requiring that trainees and fellows "pay back" their funding support by engaging in health research or teaching.

Finally, Congress decreed that National Research Service Awards be made only in areas for which "there is a need for personnel" and directed that the National Academy of Sciences provide periodic guidance on the fields in which researchers were likely to be required and on the numbers that should be trained (see Box 1-1). The present study is the eleventh to offer such guidance.

FROM 1975 TO 1994: THE FIRST TEN STUDIES

While explicit in its instruction that the number of National Research Service Awards be determined by the "national need" for biomedical and behavioral research personnel, Congress left it to those examining the workforce to define "need" and the specific fields to be considered. The earliest committee to study the subject, convened by the National Academy of Sciences in early 1975, characterized need in terms of demand for faculty, as shaped by federal support for university-based research and enrollments in higher education.[26] This committee also interpreted the term "biomedical and behavioral" as encompassing investigators in the basic biomedical sciences, the behavioral sciences, the clinical sciences, and health services research. In their first full length report, issued the following year, committee members concluded that Ph.D. production in the biomedical and behavioral sciences was more than adequate to meet existing demand.[27]

Indeed, with college enrollments leveling off and federal research expenditures growing at more modest rates than in the past, the committee called on the NIH to reduce the number of predoctoral students in the basic biomedical sciences by 10 percent and to limit postdoctoral support to existing levels. The committee recommended, furthermore, that predoctoral students in the basic biomedical sciences be supported largely

Box 1-1 National Research Service Award Act of 1974 (P.L. 93-348)

Sec. 472. (a) (3) Effective July 1, 1975, National Research Service Awards may be made for research or research training in only those subject areas for which, as determined under section 473, there is a need for personnel.

Sec. 473. (a) The Secretary shall, in accordance with subsection (b), arrange for the conduct of a continuing study to—

(a) establish (A) the Nation's overall need for biomedical and behavioral research personnel, (B) the subject areas in which such personnel are needed and the number of such personnel needed in each such area, and (C) the kinds and extent of training which should be provided such personnel;

(b) assess (A) current training programs available for the training of biomedical and behavioral research personnel which are conducted under this Act at or through institutes under the National Institutes of Health and the Alcohol, Drug Abuse, and Mental Health Administration, and (B) other current training programs available for the training of such personnel;

(c) identify the kinds of research positions available to and held by individuals completing such programs;

(d) determine, to the extent feasible, whether the programs referred to in clause (B) or paragraph (2) would be adequate to meet the needs established under paragraph (1) if the programs referred to in clause (A) of paragraph (2) were terminated; and

(e) determine what modifications in the programs referred to in paragraph (2) are required to meet the needs established under paragraph (1).

---

[26] National Research Council. *Personnel Needs and Training for Biomedical and Behavioral Research.* Washington, D.C.: National Academy of Sciences, 1975.

[27] National Research Council. *Personnel Needs and Training for Biomedical and Behavioral Research.* Washington, D.C.: National Academy of Sciences, 1976.

through training grants, reserving fellowships for postdoctorates, who were more likely to require mentoring than formal instruction in the practice of research.

In its evaluation of the behavioral science workforce, the committee found that overall Ph.D. production was in balance with the demand for faculty, but graduate schools were not providing sufficient numbers of Ph.D.s with the specialized training necessary to examine health-related research problems. The committee recommended shifting most NRSA training in the behavioral sciences from the predoctoral to the postdoctoral level. Because support for research training in the behavioral sciences was almost entirely (90 percent) directed toward graduate students at the time, the committee recognized that sudden changes in funding patterns could be disruptive and called for an "orderly tapering down of predoctoral support" until the recommended new distribution of 30 percent predoctoral and 70 percent postdoctoral training was reached. In contrast to its recommendation for the basic biomedical fields, the committee suggested that the NIH and ADAMHA devote most of their research training support in the behavioral sciences to training grants, even at the postdoctoral level, in order to encourage institutions to develop interdisciplinary approaches to training.

The committee found the clinical research workforce more difficult to evaluate, partly because it could not effectively measure the supply of physician investigators, but also because it was a more diverse group of researchers. The clinical research workforce includes not only M.D.s but also Ph.D.s, dentists, and other health care professionals. With available data pointing toward a decline in the supply of physician-investigators at the same time that demand for medical school faculty was growing, the committee concluded that a 10 percent increase in postdoctoral clinical research training was needed. Because of the importance of formal instruction in research methodology, the committee urged that the majority of this training (80 percent) be offered through training grants, rather than fellowships.

The committee also found health services research difficult to evaluate, in part because it was an emerging field but also because, like clinical research, it drew investigators from a variety of backgrounds. The committee recommended that because of the interdisciplinary nature of the field, research training be concentrated at the postdoctoral level and be provided primarily through training grants. The overall number in training was to be maintained at existing levels.

In the next five studies, conducted from 1977 to 1983, subsequent committees recognized the demand for researchers in industry, government, teaching hospitals, and other settings and incorporated employment trends in these sectors into their analyses of national need.[28-32] Yet it was not until 1985, when the biotechnology industry began to recruit significant numbers of Ph.D.s, that a committee called for additional research training in the basic biomedical sciences.[33] A second increase was recommended in the subsequent report in 1989,[34] but by 1994 demand from industry appeared to be slowing, and the committee advised that NRSA training support in the basic biomedical sciences be maintained at existing levels. The 1994 committee also called for an increase in research training in the behavioral sciences. The latter recommendation was not based on an increased demand for faculty (which was expected to grow slowly at best) but was justified in the committee's view by the "continuing gains being made by behavioral scientists in areas of national interest."[35]

Throughout the first 10 studies the supply of clinical researchers was a persistent concern. In every report, committees called for increases in clinical research training largely but not exclusively through efforts to

---

[28] Institute of Medicine. *Personnel Needs and Training for Biomedical and Behavioral Research.* Washington, D.C.: National Academy of Sciences, 1977.

[29] Institute of Medicine. *Personnel Needs and Training for Biomedical and Behavioral Research.* Washington, D.C.: National Academy of Sciences, 1978.

[30] Institute of Medicine. *Personnel Needs and Training for Biomedical and Behavioral Research, 1979 Report.* Washington, D.C.: National Academy of Sciences, 1980.

[31] Institute of Medicine. *Personnel Needs and Training for Biomedical and Behavioral Research.* Washington, D.C.: National Academy Press, 1981.

[32] Institute of Medicine. *Personnel Needs and Training for Biomedical and Behavioral Research.* Washington, D.C.: National Academy Press, 1983.

[33] Institute of Medicine. *Personnel Needs and Training for Biomedical and Behavioral Research.* Washington, D.C.: National Academy Press, 1985.

[34] National Research Council. Committee on Biomedical and Behavioral Research Personnel. *Biomedical and Behavioral Research Scientists: Their Training and Supply. Volume I: Findings.* Washington, D.C.: National Academy Press, 1989.

[35] National Research Council. *Meeting the Nation's Needs for Biomedical and Behavioral Scientists.* Washington, D.C.: National Academy Press, 1994.

attract additional numbers of physicians into research. Committees also periodically addressed the demand for investigators in health services, nursing, and dental research and generally recommended that additional opportunities for research training be offered in these areas to build up what were regarded as emerging and underutilized fields.

In the years since the NRSA program was established, funding for research training has grown much more slowly than the NIH budget,[36] a result in part of recommendations from the studies of the research workforce conducted between 1975 and 1994. When the first NRSA awards were made for research training in 1975, the program supported 14,443 students and postdoctoral fellows.[37] In 1998 the NRSA program supported 15,670 students and fellows, a number projected to increase slightly in 1999 to 15,681.[38]

To date, the NRSA program has provided research training in the biomedical and behavioral sciences to more than 130,000 students and young investigators through a combination of individual fellowship awards and institutional training grants at almost 750 universities, research institutes, and teaching hospitals.[39]

CHANGES IN THE NATIONAL RESEARCH SERVICE AWARD PROGRAM

Since its beginnings, NRSA research training has undergone a number of modifications as a result of steps taken by the Congress and the NIH, which in some cases were prompted by recommendations from committees convened by the National Academies. These actions have extended the program into new areas of research training, established funding levels for selected disciplines and educational expenses, reduced the service obligation for recipients of NRSA support, and sought to foster the recruitment of women and minorities into research careers.

The first changes in the scope of research training came in 1976, when Congress broadened the new NRSA program to encompass nursing.[40] Then, along with the NIH appropriations that year, Congress directed the administrators of the Minority Access to Research Careers program in the National Institute of General Medical Sciences to support research training for undergraduates.[41] With that mandate, the NIH began to make NRSA training available to undergraduates at historically black colleges and other minority-serving institutions. (The full array of NRSA training grants and fellowships is described in Appendix A.)

In 1978, Congress waived the service payback component of the NRSA program for those pursuing short-term training for periods up to three months.[42] The payback requirement, which had been put into place when the NRSA program began, obligated recipients to engage in a year of health research or teaching for each year of NRSA support. As soon as the requirement went into effect, however, there was a sharp decline in the number of medical and other health professions students participating in summer or other short-term training experiences. It was widely believed at the time, and substantiated by later studies,[43] that early research experience played a role in the decision to seek formal research training and pursue a research career. Therefore, the dramatic drop in participation was a cause for concern and ultimately prompted congressional action.

The scope of the program was further broadened in 1978, when Congress expanded the NRSA program to cover training in health services research[44] and again in 1985 when Congress incorporated primary care research.[45] Specific funding targets were established with the Health Research Extension Act of 1985, when Con-

[36] National Institutes of Health. Department of Health and Human Services. *NIH Data Book, 1985.* Bethesda, Md.: NIH, 1985.

[37] National Research Council. *Personnel Needs and Training for Biomedical and Behavioral Research.* Washington, D.C.: National Academy of Sciences, 1975.

[38] National Institutes of Health. Office of Financial Management. *FY 2000 Congressional Justification Overview.* Bethesda, Md.: NIH, 1998, p. 30.

[39] Unpublished tabulation from the NIH IMPAC System; on file in the archives of the Academies.

[40] *Health Research and Health Services Amendments of 1976.* P.L. 94-278, Title II, Section 201. 94th Cong., 2nd sess., 22 April 1976.

[41] U.S. Congress. Senate. Committee on Appropriations. *Departments of Labor and Health, Education, and Welfare and Related Agencies Appropriation Bill, 1977.* 94th Cong., 2nd sess., 1976. S. Rept. 94-997, p. 57.

[42] *Community Mental Health Centers Extension Act of 1978.* P.L. 95-622, 95th Cong., 2nd sess., Title II, Part D, 15 May 1978.

[43] Sherman, Charles R., H. Paul Jolly, Thomas E. Morgan, Elizabeth J. Higgins, Donald Hollander, Terry Bryll, and Ezekiel R. Sevilla. Office of Program Planning and Evaluation, National Institutes of Health. *On the Status of Medical School Faculty and Clinical Research Manpower, 1968-1990.* Washington, D.C.: Association of American Medical Colleges, 1982.

[44] *Health Services Research, Health Statistics, and Medical Technology Act of 1978.* P.L. 95-623, Section 3. 95th Cong., 2nd sess., 9 November 1978.

[45] *Health Research Extension Act of 1985.* P.L. 99-158, Title IV, Section 487. 99th Cong., 1st sess., 20 November 1985.

gress required that 0.5 percent of NRSA funds be allocated to each of the two fields.[46] The same law directed that funds for training in health services research be administered by what is now the Agency for Healthcare Research and Quality. Research training in primary care originally came under the purview of the NIH but was delegated to the Health Resources and Services Administration by Congress in 1988 after concerns were raised that the NIH was interpreting the meaning of "primary care" too broadly.[47,48] With the passage of the NIH Revitalization Act of 1993, funding levels for training in health services and primary care research were doubled (to 1 percent of the NRSA budget for each), and these two fields remain the only ones for which specific funding levels have been established by law.[49]

The 1993 legislation instituted major changes in the service payback requirement as well. With the change in the law, predoctoral trainees and fellows were no longer obligated to pay back their NRSA support. The law was further modified to limit the payback requirement for postdoctoral trainees and fellows to 12 months and to add research training to the roster of eligible activities, prompted in part by a belief that physicians and other professional doctorates who received at least two years of training are more likely to gain the skills necessary to successfully pursue research careers. As a result, a second year of NRSA-supported postdoctoral study now fulfills the obligation incurred in the first year of postdoctoral support.[50]

In response to concerns in the early 1990s about the need for more women and minorities in research, the 1993 law also directed that NRSA training be administered so as to encourage women and individuals from disadvantaged backgrounds (including racial and ethnic minorities) to pursue research careers.[51] At the same time, Congress required the NIH to ensure that women and minorities were routinely included as subjects in clinical research studies.

More recently, the NIH adopted a new approach to educational expenses associated with research training. In the 1970s and the first part of the 1980s, NIH training grants and fellowships generally covered complete tuition and fees, but by the early 1990s rising tuition costs led a number of institutes to choose to pay less than full tuition rather than cut the number of fellows and trainees. In 1996, to restore uniformity, the NIH announced a new standard for the NRSA program: It would cover 100 percent of tuition and fees up to $2,000 and 60 percent of those costs above that level.[52]

A PORTRAIT OF RESEARCH TRAINING TODAY

As illustrated in Table 1-1, NRSA training support today is almost evenly divided between graduate students and postdoctorates, is concentrated in the basic biomedical sciences (70.7 percent), and is largely provided through training grants (83.5 percent) that are awarded to institutions that then select graduate student and postdoctoral trainees.

There are significant differences in NRSA support among fields, stemming in part from the distinctive patterns of education and career development in the basic biomedical, behavioral, and clinical sciences. Training in clinical research, for example, is more likely to be provided at the postdoctoral level (71.8 percent) than that in other fields so as to build on a foundation of clinical expertise. Clinical research training is also much more likely to be supported through training grants (95.6 percent) than that in other fields, a pattern recommended in previous NRSA studies in order to encourage universities and teaching hospitals to provide instruction in methodology.

In contrast, the current pattern of NRSA research training in the behavioral sciences illustrates the challenges of changing the allocation of research training support. Though training in the behavioral sciences was

[46] Ibid.

[47] U.S. General Accounting Office. Division of Human Resources. *Medical Research: National Research Service Awards for Research in Primary Medical Care.* A report to the chairman, Subcommittee on Health and the Environment, Committee on Energy and Commerce, House of Representatives. Washington, D.C.: Government Printing Office, July 1987.

[48] *Health Omnibus Programs Extension of 1988.* P.L. 100-607, Title VI, Section 635. 100th Cong., 2nd sess., 4 November 1988.

[49] *National Institutes of Health Revitalization Act of 1993.* P.L. 103-43, Title XVI, Section 1641. 103rd Cong., 1st sess., 10 June 1993.

[50] *National Institutes of Health Revitalization Act of 1993.* P.L. 103-43, Title XVI, Section 1602. 103rd Cong., 1st sess., 10 June 1993.

[51] *National Institutes of Health Revitalization Act of 1993.* P.L. 103-43, Title XVI, Section 1601. 103rd Cong., 1st sess., 10 June 1993.

[52] "Tuition Costs on NIH NRSA Training Grant and Fellowship Awards." *NIH Guide for Grants and Contracts*, 2 February 1996. Available: http://grants.nih.gov/grants/guide/index.html.

TABLE 1-1 Distribution of Full-Time NRSA Trainees and Fellow Positions, Fiscal Year 1998

	Predoctoral	Postdoctoral	Undergraduate[a]	Total
Basic biomedical	5,399	4,211	641	10,251
MSTP[b]	824	—	—	824
Subtotal	6,223	4,211	641	11,075 (70.7%)
Behavioral	639	475	89	1,203 (7.7%)
Clinical	882	2,280	15	3,177
Health services (AHCPR)	64	55	—	119
Primary care (HRSA)	—	96	—	96
Subtotal	946	2,431	15	3,392 (21.6%)
Total	7,808 (49.8%)	7,117 (45.4%)	745 (4.8%)	15,670

	Basic Biomedical	Behavioral	Clinical	Total
Trainees				
Predoctoral	5,791	500	840	7,131
Postdoctoral	2,478	357	2,388	5,223
Undergraduate[a]	627	89	15	731
Subtotal	8,896	946	3,243	13,085 (83.5%)
Fellows				
Predoctoral	432	139	97	668
Postdoctoral	1,733	118	52	1,903
Undergraduate[a]	14	—	—	14
Subtotal	2,179	257	149	2,585 (16.5%)
Total	11,075 (70.7%)	1,203 (7.7%)	3,392 (21.6%)	15,670

[a] Receiving support through Minority Access to Research Careers or Career Opportunities in Research training grants for the undergraduate education of minority students who plan to pursue graduate studies in the biomedical or behavioral sciences.
[b] Students in the Medical Scientist Training Program for M.D.-Ph.D. training.

SOURCES: Data are from the NIH Trainee and Fellow File; the Office of Research and Review, Education, and Policy, AHRQ; and the Bureau of Health Professions, HRSA.

more evenly divided between graduate students (53.1 percent) and postdoctorates (39.5 percent) in 1998 than in the past, the shift to an emphasis on postdoctoral training recommended by previous NAS committees has not occurred.

Today the typical duration of predoctoral support is three years in the basic biomedical sciences and two years in the behavioral sciences.[53] Although NRSA policy permits trainees and fellows to receive up to five years of predoctoral funding, many NIH institutes encourage more limited appointments, with the expectation that doctoral students have opportunities to serve as research or teaching assistants during the course of their studies. Working as a research assistant is widely regarded as an important educational experience for graduate students, particularly in the basic biomedical sciences. Federal policy has long encouraged this practice by permitting investigators to employ graduate students as research assistants and to provide tuition remission as a form of compensation, as long as "there is a bona fide employer-employee relationship between the student and the institution."[54]

[53] Pion, Georgine M. Office of Extramural Research, National Institutes of Health. *The Early Career Progress of NRSA Predoctoral Trainees and Fellows*. Bethesda, Md.: NIH, 2000.

[54] Office of Management and Budget. *Circular A-21 (Revised), Cost Principles for Educational Institutions*. Washington, D.C.: OMB, 1998.

Indeed, in 1975, when Congress replaced the NIH and ADAMHA's existing research training programs with NRSA training grants and fellowships, it took little note of the support by the two agencies of other training-related activities, such as research assistantships. At the time, more than 4,700 graduate students were working as research assistants on grants from the NIH and other agencies of the Department of Health and Human Service (DHHS). The number of postdoctorates holding similar NIH- or DHHS-funded positions is not known but was probably the majority of the nearly 3,200 postdoctoral fellows in the biomedical, behavioral, and clinical sciences supported by federal research grants that year.[55] Among these were over 100 postdoctoral fellows, mostly from Western Europe, who were awarded fellowships from NIH's Fogarty International Center for study in the U.S.[56] Close to 950 newly appointed faculty members received career development awards from the agency, allowing them an opportunity to polish their research skills before becoming independent investigators.[57] In addition to those training in academic institutions, an estimated 1,000 postdoctoral fellows and clinicians were pursuing research training on the agency's Maryland campus.[58]

While the number of NRSA training grants and fellowships has grown by less than 10 percent over the past 25 years, NIH training-related activities have increased dramatically, as illustrated in Table 1-2.

Some 12,400 graduate students today work as research assistants on NIH grants, and federal grants employ more than 11,700 postdoctoral fellows in the biomedical, behavioral, and clinical sciences. The Fogarty International Center now limits its support to people from developing nations and former socialist economies, such as the countries of Central and Eastern Europe; in 1997 the center funded about 500 full-time and another 1,000 short-term students and postdoctoral fellows. Several new types of career development awards have been introduced in recent years, and altogether these awards support more than 1,600 faculty on their way to becoming independent

[55] Unpublished tabulation from the Survey of Graduate Students and Postdoctorates in Science and Engineering; on file in the archives of the Academies.

[56] Eiss, Robert. Office of International Science Policy and Analysis, Fogarty International Center, National Institutes of Health. Personal communication, February 1998.

[57] Unpublished tabulation from the NIH IMPAC System; on file in the archives of the Academies.

[58] Chen, Philip. Office of Intramural Research, National Institutes of Health. Personal communication, February 1999.

TABLE 1-2 Training-Related Activities of the NIH

	1975	1997
Graduate research assistants	4,800	12,400
Postdoctoral research associates	3,200	11,700
Recipients of career development awards	900	1,600
Participants in Fogarty International Center training programs	100	500 full-time 1,000 part-time
Postdoctoral fellows on the NIH campus	1,000	3,500

NOTES: (1) Numbers rounded to the nearest hundred; (2) these figures include all postdoctoral research associates in the biomedical, behavioral, and clinical sciences supported by federal funds and thus overestimate the NIH role in postdoctoral training.

SOURCES: Data on graduate research assistants and postdoctoral research associates are from the Survey of Graduate Students and Postdoctorates in Science and Engineering; data on career development awards are from the NIH IMPAC system; estimates of participants in Fogarty International Center training programs and NIH intramural fellows are from the FIC Office of International Science Policy and Analysis and the NIH Office of Intramural Research.

investigators. The NIH campus now hosts almost 3,500 postdoctoral fellows and clinicians for research training.[59]

Only citizens and permanent residents of the U.S. are eligible for NRSA training grants and fellowships and NIH career development awards, whereas Fogarty International Center programs are restricted to those from outside the U.S. Opportunities for research training through most other avenues are equally available to U.S. citizens and those from abroad. There are few restrictions on employment as a research assistant or postdoctoral fellow under federal grant funding, and increasing numbers of foreign graduate students and postdoctorates in the biomedical sciences and, to a lesser extent, the behavioral sciences are supported by these mechanisms.

Because of these developments, the role of NRSA training programs in the biomedical and behavioral sciences has diminished over the years. As a result, the NIH's ability to ensure that federal funds are directed where most needed has also declined.

With fewer data available, the role NRSA support plays in training clinical investigators cannot be determined as accurately as the role it plays in the basic biomedical and behavioral sciences. Because clinical research training for physicians, dentists, and doctoral-level professionals who do not hold a Ph.D. generally takes place at the postdoctoral level, two major sources of funding that support research training in the biomedical and behavioral sciences—graduate research and university teaching assistantships—are not available. Consequently, a larger fraction of those preparing for clinical research careers may depend on NRSA training grants and fellowships than their counterparts in other fields.

RECENT DEVELOPMENTS IN RESEARCH TRAINING

Since the National Research Council's 1994 report, *Meeting the Nation's Needs for Biomedical and Behavioral Scientists*,[60] the U.S. research workforce has been the focus of considerable attention and discussion and the subject of numerous national meetings, public policy studies, and congressional hearings. Much of this activity has centered on two broad areas of concern: (1) the declining numbers of health care professionals pursuing research training and careers in clinical research and (2) the growing population of Ph.D.s, particularly in the basic biomedical sciences.

A synopsis of these developments must surely begin with the 1994 "national needs" report itself and the response to the report by the NIH, the Agency for Healthcare Research and Quality, and the Health Resources and Services Administration. Of the eight principal recommendations of the committee that preceded ours, the agencies focused on two: (1) increasing the stipends for trainees and fellows and (2) evaluating the NRSA program. Since then, NRSA stipend levels have been increased three times, and the NIH has evaluated its NRSA training in the biomedical and behavioral sciences. Recommendations for expanding the number of NRSA training grants and fellowships in the behavioral and clinical sciences, oral health, nursing, and health services research were not acted on, prompting Congress to request a report on the agencies' progress in 1996. In explaining their actions to Congress, NIH, AHRQ, and HRSA officials indicated that they had focused initially on the highest-priority recommendations, and they expected to direct additional research training funds to stipends until NRSA stipend levels were comparable to other sources.[61]

Following the 1994 study on the NRSA program as a whole, several subsequent reports focused on clinical research and training. In the fall of 1994, an Institute of Medicine committee issued *Careers in Clinical Research: Obstacles and Opportunities*, which included recommendations for:

- evaluating existing clinical research training programs;
- redirecting funds to the most effective forms of clinical research training;
- emphasizing training programs resulting in an advanced degree in the evaluative sciences related to clinical research;

[59] Alexander, James. Office of Education, National Institutes of Health. Personal communication, February 1999.

[60] National Research Council. *Meeting the Nation's Needs for Biomedical and Behavioral Scientists*. Washington, D.C.: National Academy Press, 1994.

[61] National Institutes of Health. *Implementing the Recommendations in the 1994 Report from the National Academy of Sciences: Meeting the Nation's Needs for Biomedical and Behavioral Scientists*. Report to the U.S. House of Representatives, Subcommittee on Labor, Health and Human Services, and Education, Committee on Appropriations. Bethesda, Md.: NIH, 1997.

- increasing the number of M.D.-Ph.D. and D.D.S.-Ph.D. programs that train investigators with expertise in patient-oriented research; and
- expanding initiatives that reduce educational debt, through tuition subsidies, as in the case of M.D.-Ph.D. programs, and through loan forgiveness.[62]

In the spring of 1995, NIH Director Harold Varmus convened a committee to review the status of clinical research in the U.S. and consider, among other topics, the recruitment and training of future clinical researchers. The NIH Director's Panel on Clinical Research report, issued in late 1997, echoed many of the suggestions for clinical research training put forth by the Institute of Medicine.[63] Its recommendations included:

- clinical research training programs aimed at medical students, such as M.D.-Ph.D. programs for clinical research;
- ensuring that postdoctoral training grants include formal coursework or degree programs in clinical research;
- new support mechanisms for young and mid-term clinical investigators; and
- steps to reduce researchers' educational debts.

Between the time the NIH director's panel was convened and its final report, several of its suggestions for training of clinical investigators had already been adopted by the agency. In late 1996, the NIH announced a program to bring medical and dental students to its Maryland campus for a one- to two-year clinical research training experience.[64] In early 1997, the National Institute for General Medical Sciences issued new guidelines for its M.D.-Ph.D. training grants, encouraging research training in additional fields such as computer sciences, epidemiology, public health, bioengineering, biostatistics, bioethics, and economics and other social sciences.[65]

After the panel's final report in early 1998, the NIH took several additional steps to respond to the group's recommendations. First, the agency introduced three new types of career development awards: the K23 to provide health care professionals committed to clinical research careers with a period of supervised study and research;[66] the K24 to support the research and mentoring activities of mid-career clinical investigators;[67] and the K30 to provide institutions with the funds to develop or expand formal coursework in areas related to clinical research.[68] Later that year, clinical fellows at the NIH were offered the opportunity to enroll in a joint master's degree program in clinical research with Duke University.[69]

In 1995, another Institute of Medicine committee issued *Health Services Research: Workforce and Educational Issues*, which endorsed the number of training positions in health services research that had been recommended in the 1994 "national needs" study. It also encouraged the AHRQ to focus its training funds on areas in which researchers are in short supply, such as outcomes measurement, biostatistics, epidemiology, health economics, and health policy, and to provide a number of institutional training grants for innovative research training programs.[70] In 1998, the AHRQ responded to the latter recommendation by granting "innovation awards" to 10 institutions to support the design and implementation of new models of health services research training.[71]

Doctoral training in the basic biomedical sciences, and to a lesser extent, in the behavioral sciences, have also been the subject of multiple studies since 1994. In a study sponsored by the National Science Foundation

---

62 Institute of Medicine. *Careers in Clinical Research: Obstacles and Opportunities.* Washington, D.C.: National Academy Press, 1994.

63 National Institutes of Health. Director's Panel on Clinical Research. *Report to the Advisory Committee to the NIH Director.* Bethesda, Md.: NIH, 1997.

64 National Institutes of Health. Clinical Research Training Program. *Application to the National Institutes of Health Clinical Research Training Program.* Bethesda, Md.: NIH, 1996.

65 "NIGMS Guidelines for National Research Service Awards," *NIH Guide for Grants and Contracts*, 7 February 1997. Available: http://grants.nih.gov/grants/guide/index.html.

66 "Mentored Patient-Oriented Research Career Development Award," *NIH Guide for Grants and Contracts*, 6 April 1998. Available: http://grants.nih.gov/grants/guide/index.html.

67 "Midcareer Investigator Award in Patient-Oriented Research," *NIH Guide for Grants and Contracts*, 6 April 1998. Available: http://grants.nih.gov/grants/guide/index.html.

68 "Clinical Research Curriculum Award," *NIH Guide for Grants and Contracts,* 6 April 1998. Available: http://grants.nih.gov/grants/guide/index.html.

69 Campbell, Paulette Walker. "Duke U. and NIH Collaborate to Train Clinical Researchers." *Chronicle of Higher Education* 45, no. 14 (27 November 1998): A30.

70 Institute of Medicine. *Health Services Research: Work Force and Educational Issues.* Washington, D.C.: National Academy Press, 1995.

71 Agency for Health Care, Policy, and Research. *Innovation and Incentive Awards.* Rockville, Md.: AHCPR, 1998.

and Department of Energy, the Academies' Committee on Science, Engineering, and Public Policy reviewed graduate education in the biological, physical, engineering, and social sciences. In its 1995 report, *Reshaping the Graduate Education of Scientists and Engineers*, the committee called on universities to offer a broader range of academic options to their students and on federal agencies to promote this goal by supporting graduate education through training grants.[72] While it believed that research assistantships should remain an option for graduate student support, the committee recognized that an increased emphasis on training grants could reduce the number of research assistantships available. The committee also urged universities to provide better career information and guidance to students and appealed to universities, government, industry, and professional organizations to work together to develop a national human resource policy for scientists and engineers.

In response to a congressional inquiry about how it was planning to adapt its policies in the wake of *Reshaping the Graduate Education of Scientists and Engineers*, NIH indicated that, because the agency already relied heavily on training grants, its approach to funding graduate education was likely to remain much the same.[73] With regard to the other major recommendations, the NIH noted that existing training grant guidelines permitted research training in industry and other settings and pledged that it would take steps to encourage institutions with training grants to expose students to a range of career options.

Subsequently, in 1997 the National Institute of General Medical Sciences announced new guidelines for its training grants in the basic biomedical sciences and urged graduate programs to provide opportunities for internships in industry and other settings and for experience in teaching.[74] In addition, graduate programs were encouraged to supply trainees with information on career outcomes of graduates and to provide seminars and workshops on employment opportunities and career counseling.

Shortly after *Reshaping the Graduate Education of Scientists and Engineers* was published, William Massy of Stanford University and Charles Goldman of RAND released a discussion paper on the supply and demand for Ph.D.s in science and engineering.[75] The authors concluded that enrollment of doctoral students is driven more by the need for research and teaching assistants than by the labor market for Ph.D.s and that the resulting "overproduction" of Ph.D.s has led to chronic underemployment and deteriorating career attractiveness in affected fields. Consequently, increased research funding will worsen job prospects in the long run if faculty members responded by admitting more doctoral students to serve as research assistants. The authors maintained that restructuring academic research was the only sure way to bring the production of Ph.D.s into balance with demand. While improvements in the development and dissemination of data on the scientific and engineering labor markets can serve as a basis for restraining production rates, major changes in Ph.D. production will occur only when departments reduce their dependence on the research and teaching services provided by doctoral students.

A 1996 consensus conference sponsored by the Federation of American Societies for Experimental Biology addressed some of the issues raised by Massy and Goldman and objected to federal regulation of the size of graduate programs.[76] Instead, the conference report called for prospective students to be informed about employment trends in their fields of interest and for universities to "self-regulate" the size of graduate programs. Though it urged institutions to refrain from admitting graduate students in order to fulfill a need for teaching or research assistants, the conference report did not offer any advice about how those needs should otherwise be met.

In the fall of 1998, a National Research Council committee examining the career paths of young investigators also recommended restraint in the rate of growth in the number of graduate students in the life sciences.[77] In *Trends in the Early Careers of Life Sci-*

[72] National Academy of Sciences. *Reshaping the Graduate Education of Scientists and Engineers.* Washington, D.C.: National Academy Press, 1995.

[73] Harold Varmus, letter to Congressman Schiff, 30 October 1995.

[74] "NIGMS Guidelines for National Research Service Awards," *NIH Guide for Grants and Contracts*, 7 February 1997. Available: http://grants.nih.gov/grants/guide/index.html.

[75] Massy, William F., and Charles A. Goldman. *The Production and Utilization of Science and Engineering Doctorates in the United States.* Stanford Institute for Higher Education Research Discussion Paper. Stanford, Calif.: 1995.

[76] Federation of American Societies for Experimental Biology. *Graduate Education: Consensus Conference Report.* Bethesda, Md.: FASEB, 1997.

[77] National Research Council. *Trends in the Early Careers of Life Scientists.* Washington, D.C.: National Academy Press, 1998.

entists, the committee warned that the number of Ph.D.s awarded annually may already be too high and echoed the recommendations of previous reports in calling for students to be better informed about career prospects in their fields. The report also urged educators to limit the size of graduate programs in the life sciences and suggested that the federal government shift support for graduate students from research grants to training grants or fellowships.

In November of 1998, Elizabeth Marincola and Frank Solomon of the American Society for Cell Biology published an analysis of the changing career paths in cell biology and their implications for research training.[78] Drawing on the results of a 1997 survey of the society's members, the authors concluded that by every measure examined (e.g., time to degree, number of postdoctoral appointments, finding an independent position, obtaining grant funding), establishing a research career is more difficult today than in the past. In light of these findings and the high levels of dissatisfaction reported by younger members of the society—31 percent questioned their decision to get a Ph.D., reporting that they "probably" or "definitely" would not do so again—Marincola and Solomon cautioned that the future of research could be at risk if steps were not taken to lessen the barriers to a science or science-related career. Among the measures favored by the authors were adapting training to the career goals of trainees and the creation of professional research positions that do not involve teaching or grant writing.

THE CURRENT STUDY

The Committee on National Needs for Biomedical and Behavioral Scientists began its work in late 1997, in the wake of the studies, meetings, and changes in public policy detailed above. The committee's deliberations benefited a great deal from this work, as will be evident in further discussion of many of these developments throughout the report.

The committees that preceded ours in studying "national needs" for the biomedical and behavioral workforce were charged with estimating the future supply and demand for researchers and with developing recommendations for the size and other features of the NRSA program. In a departure from that approach, the NIH asked that the current committee make recommendations concerning not only the size of the NRSA program but also the overall production of research personnel. Specifically, the committee was charged with:

- estimating the current and future supply of scientists;
- estimating the future demand for scientists;
- utilizing estimates of the future demand for scientists and information about the current balance between supply and demand to develop recommendations for the appropriate size of the NRSA program and the overall production of research personnel in the biomedical, behavioral, and clinical sciences; and
- developing recommendations for improving the NRSA program.

Following an initial planning session in October of 1997, the committee of eleven experts in the fields of biomedical, behavioral, and clinical research, labor economics, and demography (see Appendix B) held four meetings to gather information on research training and draft their recommendations. During the course of its meetings, the committee heard from representatives of the NIH, AHRQ, and HRSA as well as professional societies, faculty members, and researchers in training. Comments from the interested public were also sought, through letters to 885 research and industry experts, graduate deans, directors of training programs, fellows, and trainees. The committee received 109 letters and statements in response, which are summarized in Appendix C.

The committee concentrated its attention on the three broad fields of biomedical, behavioral, and clinical research, with dental, nursing, and health services research included in the latter category. Because the last committee to consider workforce needs in these fields concluded that models of supply and demand could not be relied on for valid forecasts and suggested that future committees be guided by a demographic analysis of the research workforce, many of the current recommendations are based on the results of such a demographic analysis. This analysis considered such factors as the average age of current investigators in the biomedical and behavioral sciences, the number of Ph.D.s expected to join the workforce in the years ahead, and the likely effect of retirements and deaths. The committee supplemented this analysis by reviewing such

[78] Marincola, Elizabeth, and Frank Solomon. "The Career Structure in Biomedical Research: Implications for Training and Trainees." The American Society for Cell Biology Survey on the State of the Profession. *Molecular Biology of the Cell* 9 (November 1998): 3003-6.

indicators of short-term demand as trends in faculty and industry hiring and perceptions of the job market by recent Ph.D.s.

Chapters 2, 3, and 4 review trends in the preparation and employment of basic biomedical, behavioral, and clinical researchers and make recommendations for each field. The report concludes in Chapter 5 with an examination of minority researchers and other issues that cut across the three broad fields.

The committee regards the NRSA program as a substantial achievement, of which the NIH, the Agency for Healthcare Research and Quality, and the Health Resources and Services Administration can justifiably be proud. The committee believes, however, that the research workforce will require continuing attention and change if its successes are to continue and increase. In particular, the committee believes that the NRSA program must increase its efforts to recruit and train investigators who will address the severe and too often neglected health needs of minority populations and investigators who will integrate and translate the rapidly increasing body of knowledge of fundamental science into programs to improve the health of Americans and people around the world.

2

Basic Biomedical Scientists

DEFINING THE WORKFORCE

The basic biomedical workforce has traditionally been defined as investigators holding Ph.D.s in fields related to human health and the basic biological mechanisms that underlie health,[1] for example, biochemistry, microbiology, molecular biology, and other related disciplines listed in Appendix E. Those who graduate from universities in the U.S. with Ph.D.s in these fields and seek careers in science and engineering in this country are considered part of the basic biomedical workforce until they retire, die, or leave science and engineering for another field of work.

This definition of the basic biomedical workforce encompasses M.D.-Ph.D.s and other dual-degree holders but not scientists without a Ph.D. Although many M.D.s and other investigators holding doctoral-level professional degrees (such as veterinarians and dentists) make major contributions to the basic biomedical sciences, their numbers are difficult to estimate. We were thus unable to include them in our analysis of the size and demographic characteristics of this workforce. Nonetheless, it is important to recognize that the basic biomedical workforce includes many who have not earned Ph.D.s and that their training follows a path that differs from traditional doctoral programs in the basic biomedical sciences.

[1] National Research Council. *Meeting the Nation's Needs for Biomedical and Behavioral Scientists*. Washington, D.C.: National Academy Press, 1994.

A PORTRAIT OF THE WORKFORCE

Since 1975 the basic biomedical workforce has more than doubled in size, increasing from just over 40,600 Ph.D.s to nearly 93,000 in 1997 (see Figure 2-1). The workforce grew at a steady pace over most of this period until 1995, when its growth escalated more rapidly.

This recent growth, however, should be interpreted with caution. A change in the survey methodology in 1993 may have affected subsequent estimates of workforce size by classifying individuals by occupation (e.g., scientist, professor, manager), rather than by the scientific field in which they worked. In addition, at least part of this reported workforce growth appears to have stemmed from a change in the analysis of survey responses by the National Opinion Research Center when it took over the management of the Survey of Doctorate Recipients in 1997.

As illustrated in Figure 2-1, the growth in the overall workforce was accompanied by increasing numbers of women entering the field. Between 1975 and 1997 the number of women in the basic biomedical workforce more than quadrupled, growing from 6,529 to 27,239. By 1997 women made up 29.3 percent of the workforce, up from 16.1 percent in 1975.

The number of underrepresented minorities in the basic biomedical workforce also increased dramatically, from 1,076 in 1975 to 3,943 in 1997 (see Table G-4). Still, minorities remain a small percentage of the overall workforce. In 1997, 4.2 percent of biomedical scientists were underrepresented minorities, compared to 2.6 percent in 1975.

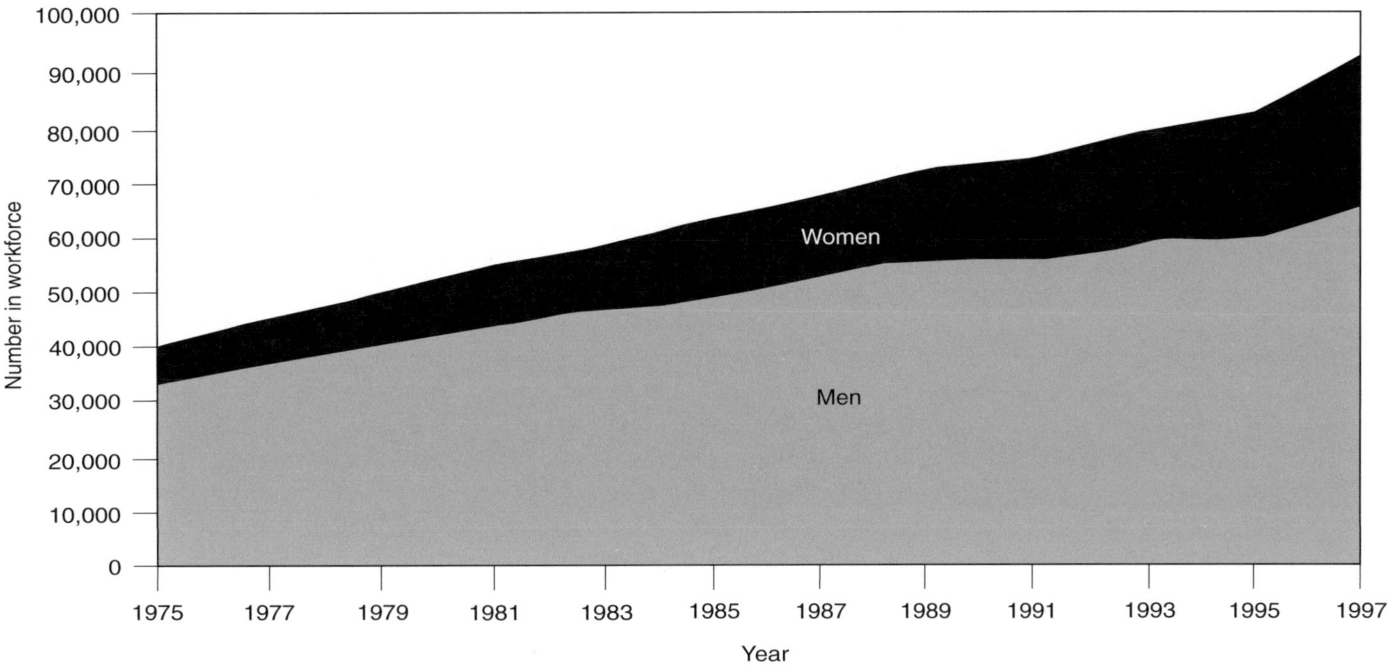

FIGURE 2-1 Gender composition of the basic biomedical workforce. SOURCE: Data are from the Survey of Doctorate Recipients (see Table G-4).

As a result of substantial increases in the numbers of Ph.D.s entering the basic biomedical workforce, the median age of the workforce has grown only modestly over the last decade, rising from 43 years in 1987 to 45.7 in 1997.[2] A demographic analysis of the workforce estimates that the median age of the basic biomedical workforce is likely to increase less than a year by 2005 to 46.2 (see Appendix D).

Unless there is a major departure from current trends in Ph.D. production and retirement, the basic biomedical workforce is projected to grow at a rate of 3.4 percent annually for the next several years. By 2005, women are expected to make up 36 percent of this workforce, which is likely to number more than 128,500 Ph.D.s.

TRENDS IN THE EDUCATION OF BASIC BIOMEDICAL SCIENTISTS

As shown in Figure 2-2, doctorate production in the basic biomedical sciences was relatively stable from 1975 to 1985 but began to increase at a rapid pace thereafter. By 1997 the number of Ph.D.s awarded in the biomedical sciences reached 5,420.

Over the course of the last two decades, the fraction of women among new Ph.D.s grew steadily, increasing from 23.9 percent overall in 1975 to 42.8 percent in 1997. International students have also become a growing component of new basic biomedical Ph.D.s. In 1975 students on temporary visas were 8.3 percent of new Ph.D.s (see Figure 2-3). By 1997 the fraction of students on temporary visas had risen to 21.6 percent.

In contrast, the proportion of underrepresented minorities earning Ph.D.s in the basic biomedical sciences has increased only gradually over the last few decades. In 1997, 4.7 percent of new Ph.D.s were from groups underrepresented in science, up from 2.4 percent in 1975. The absolute numbers represented by these percentages are small: in 1997 only 255 Ph.D.s in these fields were awarded to minorities (see Table G-1).

Between 1975 and 1990 the median time to degree in the basic biomedical sciences grew steadily from 6 years to 7.6 years, as measured from entry into postbaccalaureate study (see Table G-1). Since then the increase in time to degree has continued, though at a slower pace; Ph.D.s in 1997 spent a median of 7.8 years earning their degrees. As a result, median age at receipt

[2] Unpublished tabulation from the Survey of Doctorate Recipients; available from the archives of the Academies.

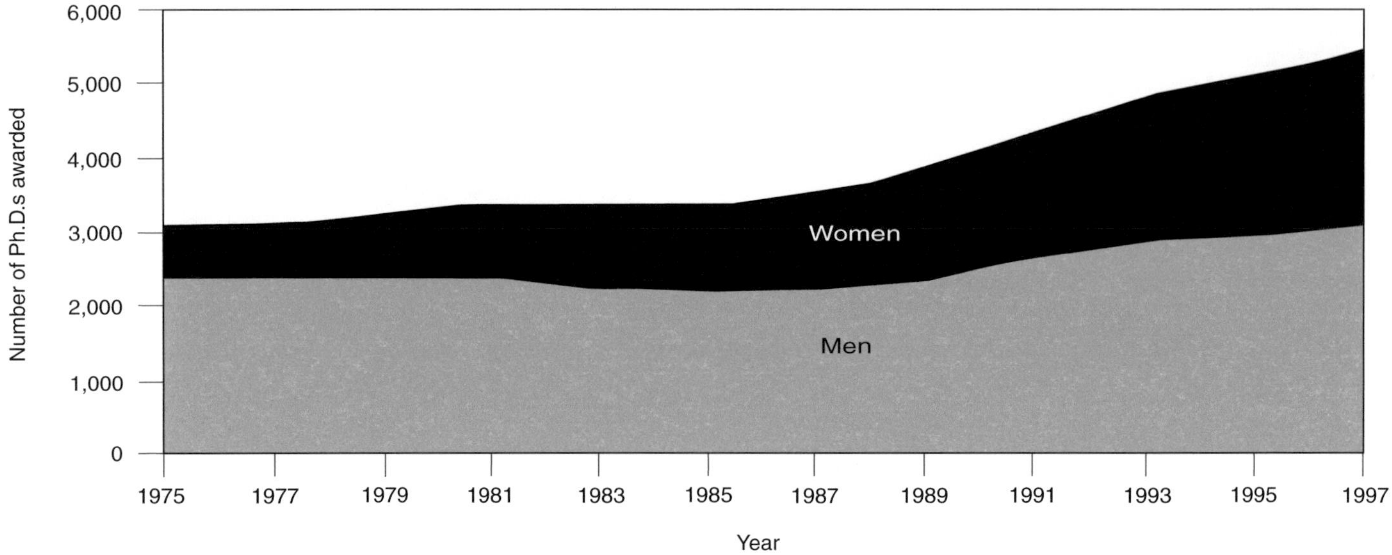

FIGURE 2-2 Ph.D.s awarded in the basic biomedical sciences in the United States by gender. SOURCE: Data are from the Survey of Earned Doctorates (see Table G-1).

of the Ph.D. also rose over this period, from 29.3 in 1975 to 30.9 in 1997.

Unlike many other fields, a period of temporary postdoctoral employment or study is a necessary step for most Ph.D.s in the basic biomedical sciences. Though the percentage of biomedical Ph.D.s planning to take a postdoctoral position after graduation has declined from its peak in 1993 (at nearly 75 percent), just over 65 percent of biomedical Ph.D.s receiving their degrees in 1997 reported plans for postdoctoral work

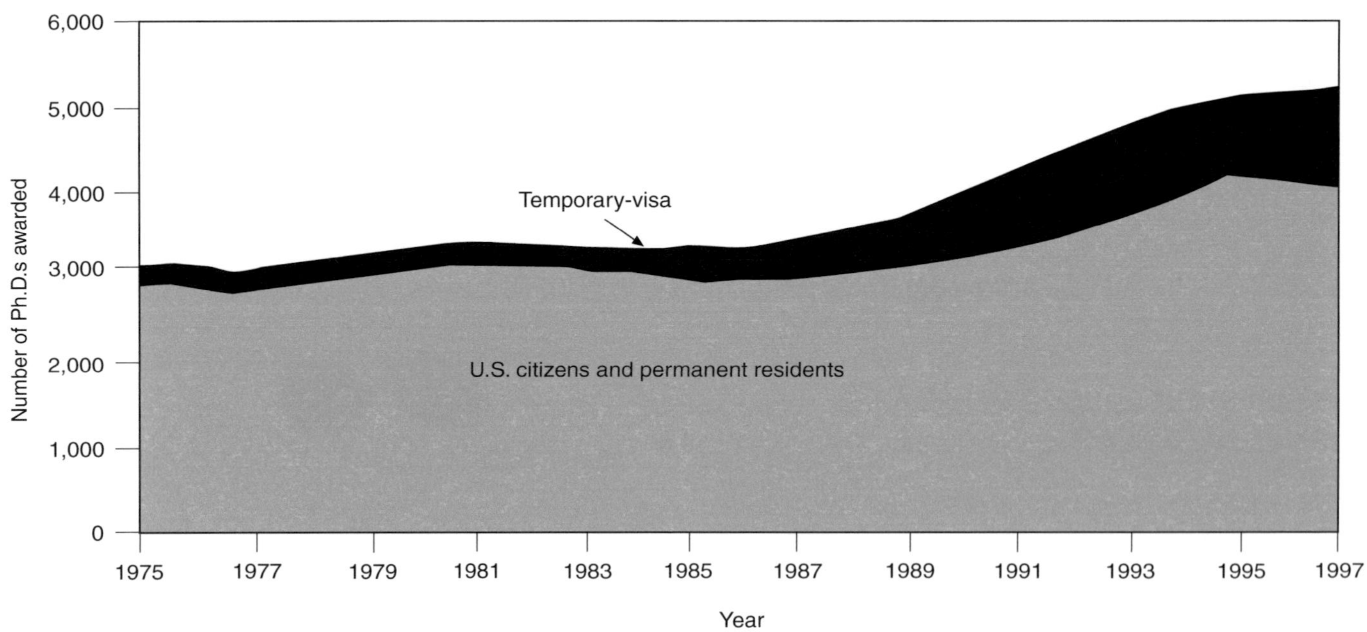

FIGURE 2-3 Ph.D.s awarded in the basic biomedical sciences in the United States by citizenship. SOURCE: Data are from the Survey of Earned Doctorates (see Table G-1).

or study (see Table G-1). Moreover, those who accept postdoctoral appointments spend increasing amounts of time in such positions. Among Ph.D.s graduating in the early 1970s who pursued postdoctoral work or study, 60.7 percent spent between two and four years in postdoctoral appointments, and 20.6 percent spent more than four years in such positions. In contrast, among Ph.D.s who received their degrees in the late 1980s and completed postdoctorates in the 1990s, 76.3 percent spent between two and four years in postdoctoral work or study and 39.8 percent spent more than four years in such appointments.[3]

TRENDS IN EMPLOYMENT

Upon completion of training, Ph.D.s in the basic biomedical sciences have traditionally worked in academic settings, and that remains the case for the majority of those in the workforce today. For the purposes of this analysis, those holding postdoctoral appointments are considered to be in the workforce and those who are self-employed are classified as working in industry. Over the last two decades, however, increasing numbers of basic biomedical scientists have pursued job opportunities in industry, and nearly one-quarter of the biomedical workforce can now be found in industrial settings (see Figure 2-4).

From 1975 to 1997 the number of biomedical scientists working in industry more than quadrupled (from 5,326 to 22,204) and the fraction of the biomedical workforce in that sector rose from 13.1 percent to 23.9 percent. The number of biomedical scientists in academia also grew but at a much more gradual pace, from 27,219 in 1975 to 53,026 in 1997. As a result, the portion of basic biomedical Ph.D.s working in academic settings dropped from 67 percent in 1975 to 57 percent in 1997. Over the same time period, biomedical scientists working in government more than doubled in number, rising to 8,649 in 1997; government scientists now represent 9.3 percent of the biomedical workforce.

While industrial employment has increased nationally, opportunities for such work vary widely by region. In 1997, for example, 65.2 percent of biomedical scientists working in New Jersey were employed in industry. The same was true of 39.3 percent of biomedical Ph.D.s working in Connecticut and 37.5 percent of those working in California. In Maryland, however, where the National Institutes of Health (NIH) and other

[3] Unpublished tabulation from the Survey of Earned Doctorates; available from the archives of the Academies.

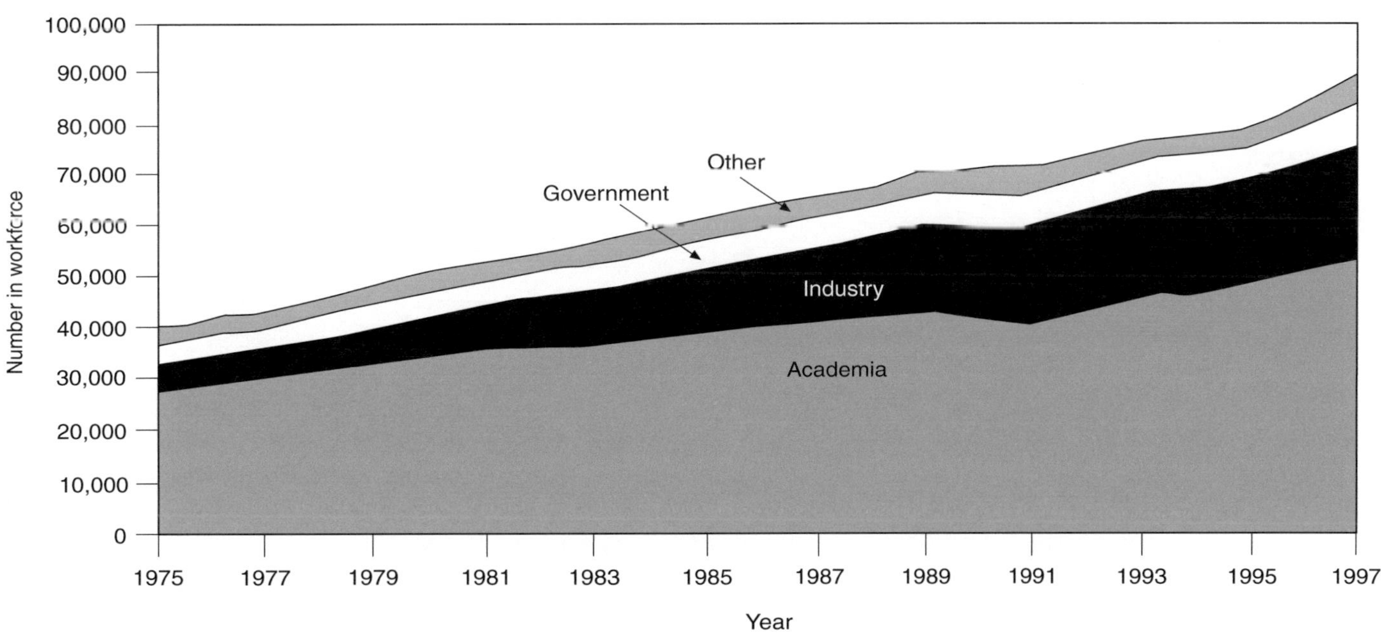

FIGURE 2-4 Employment of basic biomedical scientists by sector. SOURCE: Data are from the Survey of Doctorate Recipients (see Table G-4).

federal laboratories are the major employer, only 14.1 percent of biomedical Ph.D.s were employed in industry.[4]

Since the mid-1990s, the rate of growth in industrial employment has slowed. After steadily increasing throughout the 1980s and early 1990s, the overall fraction of biomedical scientists working in industry peaked at 25.1 percent in 1993. Subsequent reductions in the pace of hiring caused a modest decline in the fraction of the biomedical workforce employed in industry, which registered 23.9 percent in 1997.

In academic settings, where most biomedical Ph.D.s continue to find employment, the types of positions common today are markedly different from those available two decades ago. As shown in Figure 2-5, nearly all (81.7 percent) biomedical Ph.D.s in academia in the mid-1970s were tenured or tenure-track faculty members. Only 9.6 percent of biomedical Ph.D.s in academic institutions were employed in postdoctoral positions. By 1997, however, the fraction of biomedical Ph.D.s in academia who were tenured or were on tenure track had dropped to 55.3 percent, and those in postdoctoral positions had risen to 18.1 percent. Over the same period, the number of nontenure-track faculty increased more than tenfold, so that by 1997, 12.9 percent of biomedical Ph.D.s in academic institutions held such appointments. In addition, "other academic" positions (such as research associates and instructors) more than quadrupled in number, rising from 6.3 percent of the academic workforce in 1975 to 13.8 percent in 1997.

National surveys of the Ph.D. workforce supply less detail about the types of jobs held by government scientists, but the growth in postdoctorates in that sector has followed the same upward trend as in academia. From 1975 to 1997, the fraction of biomedical Ph.D.s employed in government who held postdoctoral positions increased from 6.1 to 16.6 percent (see Table G-4). Postdoctorates increased in industry as well but remained well below the levels found in government and academia: only 2.5 percent of biomedical Ph.D.s working in industry reported holding postdoctoral appointments in 1997.

As is the case for all highly educated workers, unemployment rates for Ph.D.s consistently register well below the overall national average, and biomedical scientists are no exception. In 1997 just 1.2 percent of biomedical Ph.D.s were unemployed.[5] The same year

[4] Unpublished tabulation from the Survey of Doctorate Recipients; available from the archives of the Academies.

[5] Ibid.

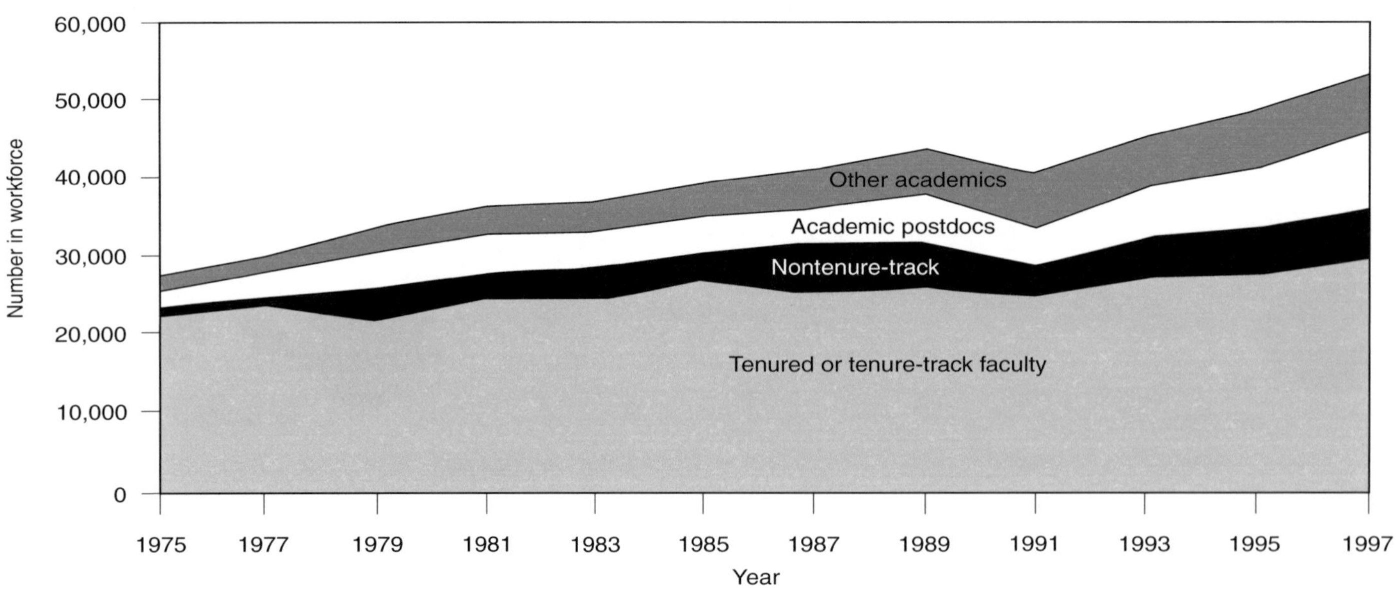

FIGURE 2-5 Employment of basic biomedical scientists in academia. SOURCE: Data are from the Survey of Doctorate Recipients (see Table G-4).

the fraction of new Ph.D.s planning postdoctoral study dropped to 65.1 percent, possibly signaling improved employment opportunities for newly minted Ph.D.s.

At the same time, there are signs that new Ph.D.s in the biomedical sciences continue to have difficulties finding suitable employment and establishing themselves professionally. Surveys conducted by microbiology and physiology societies found that more than 75 percent of newly minted Ph.D.s worked in postdoctoral or other temporary positions, and more than 40 percent reported doing so only because a suitable permanent position was not available.[6] The surveys of microbiologists found that more than twice as many Ph.D.s graduating in 1996 and 1997 viewed the job market as "bad" or "hopeless" (41 percent) than "good" or "excellent" (17 percent).[7] If they had to do it over again, 31 percent of those earning doctorates in cell biology in the 1990s reported that they "probably" or "definitely" would not pursue a Ph.D.[8]

The views of recent Ph.D.s responding to these surveys in regard to their profession and employment prospects highlight the consequences of changes in the conduct of science and the nature of its job market over the last few decades. Because the biomedical research agenda is increasingly dominated by questions that depend on teams of research personnel, many who were attracted to science for the opportunity to be "independent investigators" may find the field less satisfying than in the past.

With increasing numbers of new Ph.D.s entering the job market over the last decade and a half and comparatively few openings for independent investigators on university and medical school faculties and in government labs, Ph.D.s have increasingly taken on the day-to-day work of research—tasks that command lower salaries and in past years were often performed by technicians. This trend was noted in a 1993 study of staffing patterns for NIH grants, in which agency analysts found that "technical" and "other" support staff declined from fiscal years 1983 to 1990, while the role played by (less expensive) postdoctorates and graduate research assistants increased.[9] Consequently, some observers believe that biomedical research has two distinct job markets: one for independent investigators for whom demand is low and one for low-paid research workers for whom demand is high.

As part of the demographic analysis conducted for the committee, estimates were made of the number of graduates that would be needed from 1996 to 2005 if the biomedical research workforce grew at the same rate as the U.S. labor force as a whole (see Table D-7). Under those circumstances, the number of new biomedical science Ph.D.s that would have been needed in 1997 was estimated at 1,571—less than one-third of the actual number that year (5,420). As a result of increasing retirements and other departures from the workforce, the annual number of new Ph.D.s that will be needed is projected to rise to 3,031 by 2005. That figure still falls well below current levels of Ph.D. production.

THE ROLE OF PHYSICIANS IN THE WORKFORCE

Though often overlooked in assessments of this workforce, physician-scientists play an important role in basic biomedical research. In 1997, for example, more than one-fifth of NIH research grants for nonclincal research were awarded to M.D.s (18.2 percent) or M.D.-Ph.D.s (4.1 percent). In fact, since the NIH began to classify clinical research awards in 1996, it has become evident that both M.D.s and M.D.-Ph.D.s supported by the agency are more likely to conduct nonclinical than clinical research (see Table 4-1). Because many physician-investigators approach nonclinical research with the goal of understanding the mechanisms underlying a particular disease or disorder, their findings are often essential to improvements in human health.

Beyond the pool of NIH-funded investigators, information about the M.D. portion of the health research workforce is more difficult to obtain than about Ph.D.s (who are the subject of several national surveys sponsored by the National Science Foundation). The only data available on the national supply of physicians in

[6] Commission on Professionals in Science and Technology. *Employment of Recent Doctoral Graduates in S&E: Results of Professional Society Surveys.* Washington, D.C.: CPST, 1998.

[7] American Society for Microbiology. *Profile of Recent Doctoral Graduates in Microbiology: 1996 and 1997 Graduates.* Washington, D.C.: ASM, 1999.

[8] Marincola, Elizabeth, and Frank Solomon. "The Career Structure in Basic Biomedical Research: Implications for Training and Trainees." *Molecular Biology of the Cell* 9 (November 1998): 3003-6.

[9] National Institutes of Health, Office of Science Policy and Legislation. *Staffing Patterns of the National Institutes of Health Research Grants.* Bethesda, Md.: NIH, 1993.

research are collected by the American Medical Association, but they reveal little about the type of research conducted or whether it is carried out in a medical school, industry, or government laboratory.

According to the American Medical Association, the number of physicians active in research rose throughout the late 1970s and early 1980s and reached 22,945 by 1985.[10] Since then, however, the number of M.D.s and M.D.-Ph.D.s identifying research as their primary professional activity has steadily declined, dropping to 14,434 in 1997. If the fraction of this national pool of physician-investigators focusing on nonclinical research is similar to that supported by the NIH (66 percent), the basic biomedical workforce would have included 9,526 M.D.s and M.D.-Ph.D.s in 1997.

Though these data do not distinguish between physician-investigators holding the M.D. degree and those with M.D.-Ph.D.s, it is likely that an increasing proportion of physician-scientists hold two degrees. Since the first formal M.D.-Ph.D. training programs were introduced in 1964, opportunities for dual-degree training have steadily increased, and in 1998, 116 medical schools offered their students an opportunity to earn both degrees.[11,12] Because M.D.-Ph.D. investigators are more likely to concentrate on nonclinical research than M.D.s (see Table 4-1), this group can be expected to play an increasing role in the basic biomedical workforce in the years ahead.

As described in more detail in Chapter 4, many dual-degree students receive research training support from the NIH through National Research Service Award (NRSA) training grants and fellowships dedicated to M.D.-Ph.D. training. In addition, a number of medical schools support dual-degree training with funds from private or other sources.

On completion of their training, most M.D.-Ph.D.s enter the job market on better financial footing and with better job prospects than investigators with only one degree. Overall indebtedness levels reported by M.D.-Ph.D.s are about half those of their medical school classmates (see Table 4-3). Moreover, unlike their counterparts with a Ph.D., who often have difficulty obtaining faculty positions, M.D.-Ph.D.s are reportedly in great demand as medical school faculty members, particularly in clinical departments.

Despite such advantages, M.D.-Ph.D.s are subject to some of the same economic pressures as other medical school faculty. In competitive health care markets, they—like other junior faculty surveyed in a 1997 assessment of the activities of medical school faculty—may be more apt to be assigned to patient care duties and less likely to conduct research.[13] Indeed, by the latter half of the 1990s, M.D.-Ph.D.s emerging from some of the best-known training programs in the country were reporting difficulties identifying faculty positions that would allow them to perform research.[14]

THE CHANGING ROLE OF THE NATIONAL RESEARCH SERVICE AWARD PROGRAM

When the NRSA program began in 1975, 20,522 graduate students in the basic biomedical sciences received some form of financial assistance for their studies (see Figure 2-6). Of these, 42.9 percent (8,797) received federal funding, and more than half of those students (57.6 percent) were supported by NIH or other DHHS training grants and fellowships.

By 1997 the situation had changed dramatically. The overall number of graduate students receiving financial support in the basic biomedical sciences increased by two-thirds, to 33,873. Of these, the percentage supported by federal sources remained roughly the same (at 44.9 percent), but only 25.9 percent received funds from NIH or other DHHS training grants and fellowships. In 1997 nearly half (48.9 percent) of federal support to graduate students in the biomedical sciences took the form of research assistantships provided through NIH or other DHHS grants; another 25.1 percent of students received funds from other federal sources. In short, in just over two decades the pattern of federal support for graduate education in the biomedical sciences changed dramatically: the percentage of students receiving funds from NIH or other DHHS

[10] Pasko, Thomas, and Bradley Seidman. *Physician Characteristics and Distribution in the US, 1999*. Chicago: American Medical Association, 1999.

[11] National Institutes of Health, National Institute of General Medical Sciences. *The Careers and Professional Activities of Graduates of the NIGMS Medical Scientist Training Program*. Bethesda, Md.: NIH, September 1998.

[12] Association of American Medical Colleges. *Medical School Admissions Requirements, 2000-2001*. Washington, D.C.: AAMC, 1999.

[13] Campbell, Eric G., Joel S. Weissman, and David Blumenthal. "Relationship Between Market Competition and the Activities and Attitudes of Medical School Faculty." *JAMA* 278, no. 3 (1997): 222-26.

[14] Ledger, Kate. "Specialists for Hire." *Hopkins Medical News* (Spring-Summer 1996): 21-27.

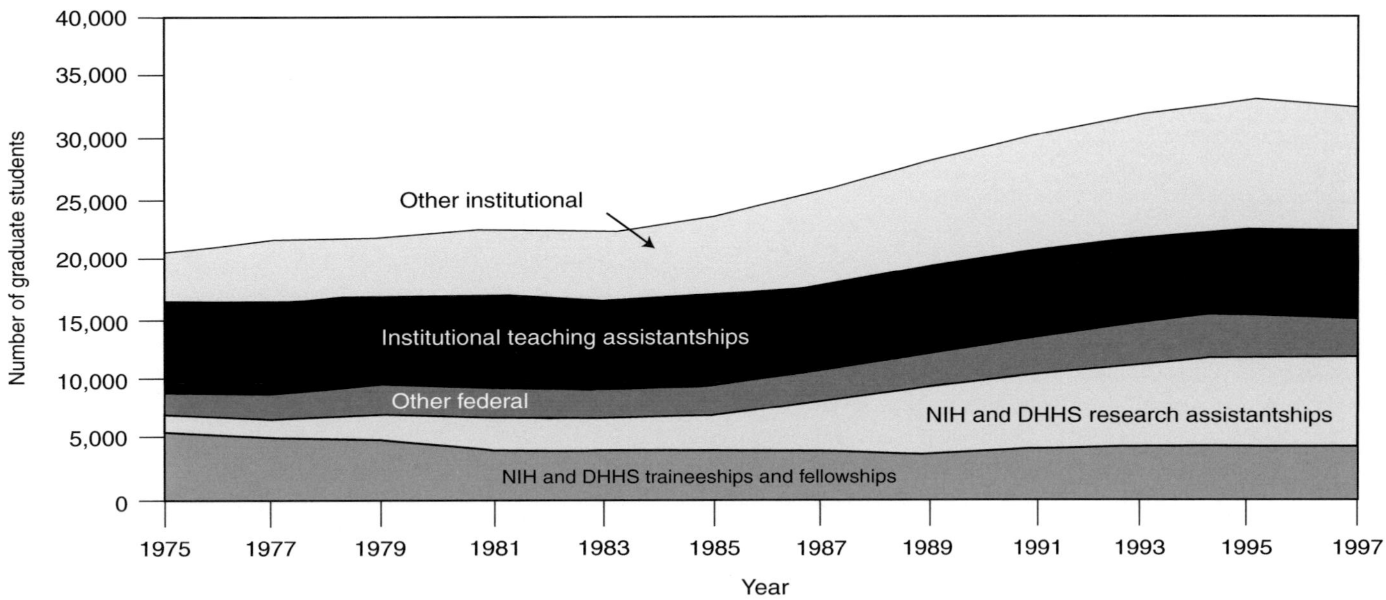

FIGURE 2-6 Trends in graduate students' primary source of support in the biomedical sciences. SOURCE: Data are from the Survey of Graduate Students and Postdoctorates in Science and Engineering (see Table G-7).

training grants and fellowships fell by more than half, while the percentage receiving funding through NIH or other DHHS research grants more than doubled.

Though the information available on funding patterns for postdoctorates in the basic biomedical sciences is much less detailed than that for graduate students, it is evident that the portion of federal funds devoted to training grants and fellowships has diminished at the postdoctoral level as well.[15] In the mid-1970s, 4,250 (77.2 percent) of the 5,506 university-based postdoctorates received federal funding for their training. Of these, 45.8 percent had federal fellowships or training grant appointments and 54.2 percent were employees on federal research grants. By 1997 the fraction of the 14,197 university-based postdoctorates receiving federal funds had declined slightly (to 71.9 percent), and a significant shift in the pattern of support had occurred. Of the 10,213 postdoctorates supported by federal funds that year, 22.3 percent had fellowships or training grant appointments, while 77.7 percent worked on research grants.

The source of this shift in the pattern of federal research training support can be found traced to a number of related trends. Over the last 25 years the number of research grants awarded by the NIH and other DHHS agencies has more than doubled.[16] Principal investigators have come to depend on graduate students and postdoctorates to carry out much of the day-to-day work of research. During the same period, both the number of universities awarding Ph.D.s in the basic biomedical sciences and the quantity of Ph.D.s awarded by existing programs have grown.[17] Federal funding policies, furthermore, have inadvertently provided universities an incentive to appoint students and postdoctorates to research assistantships instead of training grants or fellowships. As shown in Table 2-1, the NIH provides almost $9,000 more to research assistants and their institutions (largely in the form of indirect cost payments to universities) than to NRSA trainees or fellows.

As described in Chapter 1, the number of students and postdoctorates provided research training through NRSA training grants and fellowships has been deliberately limited over much of the last 25 years to ensure that the supply of investigators trained through the program would not exceed what the research enterprise could absorb. No similar federal effort has been under-

[15] Unpublished tabulation from the Survey of Graduate Students and Postdoctorates in Science and Engineering; available from the archives of the Academies.

[16] Unpublished tabulation from the NIH IMPAC System; available from the archives of the Academies.

[17] Unpublished tabulation from the Survey of Earned Doctorates; available from the archives of the Academies.

TABLE 2-1 Comparison of the Average Benefits Provided to NRSA Recipients and NIH-Supported Graduate Research Assistants, Fiscal Year 1999

NRSA Recipient		Graduate Research Assistant[a]	
Stipend	$14,688	Base salary	$16,000
Tuition benefit	8,600	Tuition reimbursement	8,400
Institutional allowance	1,500	Fringe benefits	1,600
Indirect costs	1,310	Indirect costs	8,800
Travel allowance	500		
Total cost	$26,598	Total cost	$34,800

NOTE: Comparison is based on the following assumptions:

- The average salary of graduate research assistants is $16,000.
- The fringe benefit rate for graduate research assistants is 10 percent.
- The average indirect cost rate for research grants is 50 percent and for NRSA training grants and fellowships is 8 percent.
- Institutions receive a $1,500 allowance for each predoctoral trainee; NRSA recipients may accrue some benefit from this allowance.
- The NRSA tuition benefit equals 100 percent of the first $2,000 and 60 percent of costs above $2,000; amount shown assumes that the average combined cost of tuition, fees, and health insurance is $13,000.

[a] Direct costs are capped at $26,000.

SOURCE: Data are from the NIH Office of Extramural Research.

taken thus far to ensure an adequate supply of technically prepared support staff in research, nor is there a system for regulating the number of research assistantships. Hence, as Massy and Goldman concluded in their 1995 analysis of science and engineering Ph.D. production, the size of doctoral programs is driven largely by departmental needs for research and teaching assistants, rather than by the labor market for Ph.D.s.[18]

Despite the shift in federal support, the fraction of eligible students in the biomedical sciences who receive NRSA funding during their predoctoral years has remained relatively constant over the last few decades. At some point during their training, one-third of qualifying doctoral students receive NRSA support.[19] The explanation for this seeming contradiction can be found in the eligibility requirements for NRSA awards: only U.S. citizens and permanent residents qualify for NRSA training grants and fellowships, and their number has grown at a much slower pace than that of foreign students pursuing degrees in the biomedical sciences.

This shift in the pattern of federal research training support may have long-term implications, as a result of several factors. Predoctoral NRSA training grants in the basic biomedical sciences generally take a "multidisciplinary" approach to research training, and students without benefit of such exposure may be limited in their future research activities. Moreover, evaluations of the NRSA program suggest that its participants complete their training faster than other students and go on to more productive research careers.

Since the beginning of the NRSA program, the NIH has required most predoctoral training grants in the basic biomedical sciences to be "multidisciplinary" in order to expose students to a range of biomedical fields. Though the effectiveness of multidisciplinary training undoubtedly varies from program to program, a training grant with the declared purpose of multidisciplinary training is more likely to achieve that goal than a research assistantship.

In the committee's view, the tradition of multidisciplinary training in the biomedical sciences has been valuable and could be fruitfully extended to a wider range of related fields. In spite of the efforts of

[18] Massy, William F., and Charles A. Goldman. *The Production and Utilization of Science and Engineering Doctorates in the United States.* Stanford Institute for Higher Education Research Discussion Paper. Stanford, Calif.: 1995.

[19] Unpublished tabulation from the Survey of Earned Doctorates and NIH Trainee and Fellow File; available from the archives of the Academies.

several targeted NRSA research training programs to encourage universities to integrate training in physics, chemistry, or mathematics with biology, the committee believes that too few doctoral students in the basic biomedical sciences have the opportunity to develop the breadth of knowledge that will allow them to interact effectively with investigators in related fields. Building on the rapidly increasing knowledge of molecular biology and genetics, for example, often requires work in fields outside the basic biomedical sciences. Similarly, the translation of basic biomedical discoveries into clinical applications may require collaborating with physicians and a working knowledge of such aspects of human biology as anatomy, physiology, and pharmacology.

The committee recognizes the challenge of expanding the breadth of research training without increasing time to degree, but progress in health research will be accelerated if basic biomedical scientists can readily relate their knowledge to other fields, including chemistry, mathematics, clinical medicine, and behavior. Examples of model approaches to research training that could be adopted more widely include the "Frontiers in Interdisciplinary Biosciences" course introduced at Stanford University in the fall of 1999, which brings together students from the biosciences, chemistry, physics, and engineering to evaluate cutting-edge research,[20] and the long-standing pathobiology course at the Tufts University Sackler School of Graduate Biomedical Sciences, which provides non-physician graduate students and postdoctoral fellows with grounding in human disease and the skills to collaborate with physicians.[21]

Evaluations of career outcomes suggest that NRSA participants complete training faster and go on to more successful research careers than classmates at the same institution or those graduating from universities without NRSA funding. The first of these assessments, completed in 1984, found that participants in NIH training programs completed their doctoral degrees faster and were more likely to go on to NIH-supported postdoctoral training than their counterparts who received funding from other mechanisms.[22] Moreover, those supported by the NIH during their predoctoral studies received NIH research grants more often, authored more articles, and were cited more frequently by their peers.

A more recent evaluation, conducted in the late 1990s, reported similar findings (see Figure 2-7). Basic biomedical Ph.D.s who received NRSA support for at least one academic year spent less time in graduate school. Nearly 57 percent of NRSA trainees and fellows received their doctorates by age 30, an accomplishment matched by 39 percent of their classmates and 32 percent in departments without NRSA support.[23]

After completing their studies, NRSA trainees and fellows were more likely to move into faculty or other research-intensive positions. Seven to eight years after receiving their degrees, 37 percent of former NRSA recipients held faculty appointments at institutions ranking in the top 100 in NIH funding. The same was true for 24 percent of their classmates without NRSA support and 16 percent of graduates from departments without NRSA funding. As a whole, 87 percent of former NRSA trainees and fellows reported that they were in research-related positions, in academia, industry, or other settings, compared to 77 percent of their former classmates and 72 percent of those from departments without NRSA support.

Former NRSA trainees and fellows were more likely to be successful in competing for grants. Of the 1981-1988 Ph.D. recipients who applied for NIH research grant support by 1994, the success rates were 67 percent for NRSA recipients, 55 percent for their former classmates, and 47 percent for those who graduated from departments without NRSA funding. Moreover, former trainees and fellows who completed their degrees in 1981-1982 had a median of eight and one-half publications by 1995, twice as many as Ph.D.s who graduated from departments without NRSA support, and much more than their former classmates, who published a median of five publications.

Such findings, of course, do not address the reasons

[20] Stanford University. Department of Biological Sciences. "Frontiers in Interdisciplinary Biosciences." Online. Stanford University. Available: http://cmgm.stanford.edu/biochem/biox/course.html. Accessed 23 February 2000.

[21] Arias, Irwin M. "Training Basic Scientists to Bridge the Gap Between Basic Science and Its Applications to Human Disease." *New England Journal of Medicine* 321, no. 14 (1989): 972-74.

[22] Coggeshall, Porter, and Prudence Brown. *The Career Achievements of NIH Predoctoral Trainees and Fellows*. Washington, D.C.: National Academy Press, 1984.

[23] Pion, Georgine, M. Office of Extramural Research, National Institutes of Health. *The Early Career Progress of NRSA Predoctoral Trainees and Fellows.* Bethesda, Md.: NIH, 2000.

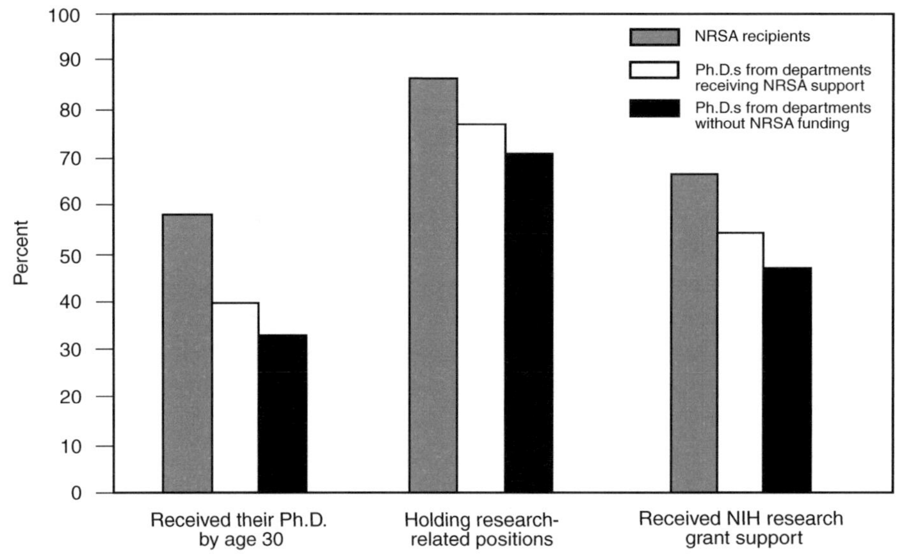

FIGURE 2-7 Selected career outcomes of basic biomedical Ph.D. recipients from 1981 to 1992 by nature of support. SOURCE: Data are from the NIH Office of Extramural Research, *The Early Career Progress of NRSA Predoctoral Trainees and Fellows,* 2000.

for the success of former NRSA trainees and fellows. The extent to which the differences in their educational and career outcomes reflect the foresight of training grant directors and fellowship reviewers in selecting the most promising candidates for NRSA funding and to what degree the outcomes are due to the training itself—or other factors—are not known. Nonetheless, it is clear that more NRSA participants go on to active and successful research careers.

IMPLICATIONS AND RECOMMENDATIONS

On the whole, the size of the basic biomedical workforce appears more than sufficient to meet national needs, and current levels of research training may be even higher than necessary to maintain the workforce. While the committee believes there are some areas of research training that should expand, overall Ph.D. production in biomedical sciences should not.

In light of the findings from the demographic analysis of the workforce conducted for the committee, some might suggest that the number of Ph.D.s awarded in biomedical science fields be reduced. Given the central role that graduate students and postdoctorates play in the conduct of basic biomedical research, however, a decrease in Ph.D. production could delay or disrupt research progress. Before considering any cutbacks, university administrators and federal policymakers must begin to address the ongoing demand for research support staff. The "nonreplicating" Ph.D.-level scientist (i.e., one who neither applies for grants nor trains students) proposed by Marincola and Solomon is one potential solution;[24] a permanent laboratory workforce of master's-level technicians and Ph.D.-trained research associates, as proposed by the NRC committee that prepared the 1998 report *Trends in the Early Careers of Life Scientists,* is another.[25]

Several steps should be taken to improve the quality of research training in the basic biomedical sciences. The committee believes that the tradition of multidisciplinary NRSA training would be even more effective if it were broadened to emphasize the connections between the biomedical sciences and other related fields. In addition, the committee is greatly concerned that the number of underrepresented minorities earning Ph.D.s in the biomedical sciences has increased at a very slow pace.

---

[24] Marincola, Elizabeth, and Frank Solomon, "The Career Structure in Basic Biomedical Research: Implications for Training and Trainees." *Molecular Biology of the Cell* 9 (November 1998): 3003-6.

[25] National Research Council. Trends in the Early Careers of Life Scientists. Washington, D.C.: National Academy Press, 1998.

Because of the successful career outcomes of its participants and its tradition of multidisciplinary training, the NRSA program should play a greater role in NIH's portfolio of research training and training-related activities than it does today. It is unlikely, however, that the NIH could readily return to its pattern of research training support of the mid-1970s, when the NRSA program was initiated and more than 70 percent of graduate students in the biomedical sciences with NIH or other DHHS support received funding through training grants or fellowships. Instead, the committee believes that the agency should strive for a middle ground: gradually expanding the NRSA program until it accounts for at least 50 percent of the agency's funding for graduate students in the basic biomedical sciences and correspondingly limiting research assistantships and other modes of graduate student support, to ensure that overall Ph.D. production does not increase. At the postdoctoral level, the NIH should also seek to provide advanced research training to a greater number of recent Ph.D.s through NRSA training grants and fellowships, rather than postdoctoral appointments on research grants.

Coordinating reciprocal increases in the NRSA program and reductions in other funding for graduate student support will undoubtedly require the NIH to consolidate its oversight of research training and training-related activities. Such a change in NIH policy and practice will also have implications for the ways in which universities administer federal research training funds, perhaps requiring more centralized control over graduate student enrollment. Moreover, if eligibility requirements for NRSA training grants and fellowships remain unchanged, a reduction in other forms of training-related support will likely reduce the number of foreign students seeking biomedical science Ph.D.s in the U.S. These and related issues are discussed in greater detail in Chapter 5.

Recommendation 2-1. There should be no growth in the aggregate number of Ph.D.s awarded in the basic biomedical sciences.

Given the current employment opportunities for basic biomedical scientists and the forecasted growth in the workforce, the present number of approximately 5,400 new basic biomedical Ph.D.s a year is more than sufficient to fulfill anticipated national needs at least until 2005.

Recommendation 2-2. Support for NRSA training grants and fellowships at the predoctoral and postdoctoral levels should be gradually increased. At the predoctoral levels, the NIH should seek to provide at least 50 percent of its research training support through training grants and fellowships.

The evidence suggests that training grants and fellowships are more effective in research career development than are research assistantships. Therefore, we recommend a gradual expansion in the numbers of students and postdoctorates supported in this fashion but only if accompanied by a concomitant decrease in training by research grants.

NIH and other federal sponsors of research training should consider options to assist graduate departments in restricting overall expansion of Ph.D. programs, including (1) encouraging universities to provide all entering graduate students with some form of financial support, such as a traineeship, that would allow them an opportunity for broad multidisciplinary education, (2) requiring graduate students to pass their qualifying exams before working as research assistants on federally funded projects, and (3) limiting the number of years graduate students may be employed as research assistants and postdoctorates may be employed in temporary appointments with federal funds.

Recommendation 2-3. The NIH should consider at least a small increase in dual-degree training in the basic biomedical sciences.

Because of the considerable success of the NRSA dual-degree training programs that prepare physicians to conduct basic biomedical research, we urge the NIH to consider at least a small increase in such programs. If it opts to expand dual-degree training, the NIH should assess the need for proportionate reductions in other forms of research training support, in order to prevent an increase in overall Ph.D. production in the basic biomedical sciences.

Recommendation 2-4. The NIH should expand its emphasis on multidisciplinary training in the basic biomedical sciences.

Since the NRSA program began, training grant awards in the basic biomedical sciences have emphasized multidisciplinary research training. Given current opportunities for basic biomedical Ph.D.s and continuing advances in science, the NIH should build on its tradition of multidisciplinary training by providing more students and fellows with the skills that will allow them to collaborate effectively with investigators in clinical medicine, the behavioral sciences, and such fields as mathematics, physics, and chemistry.

Recommendation 2-5. The NIH should increase its efforts to identify and support programs that encourage and prepare underrepresented minority students for careers in basic biomedical research.

Although there has been some increase in minority Ph.D.s in the basic biomedical sciences, their number is still low. The cause of this is likely not in graduate training but far earlier in the educational careers of students. There is a great need to evaluate and identify what works, which environments are especially successful, and where NIH interventions could make a difference.

3

Behavioral and Social Scientists

DEFINING THE WORKFORCE

Past studies of research training needs in the behavioral sciences relevant to health generally defined the target workforce as Ph.D.s trained in psychology, anthropology, sociology, and the speech and hearing sciences. The specific details of that definition have varied: some analyses have focused on psychologists trained in the nonclinical subfields of psychology (such as developmental and physiological psychology), because these individuals are more likely to be involved in research;[1] others included all Ph.D.s in psychology.[2]

Identifying the workforce of interest is further complicated by the range of research undertaken by behavioral scientists. In the basic biomedical sciences, the majority of the workforce conducts health-related research, but Ph.D.s trained in the behavioral sciences carry out a broad range of research, often unrelated to health and medicine. There is no way to identify or even estimate the numbers of Ph.D.s in the behavioral science workforce who focus on health-related research. Yet this sector of the behavioral workforce plays a critical role. Behavior is increasingly recognized as a key element both in the maintenance of good health and the development of disease. When illness occurs, a patient's behavior often affects the efficacy of treatment and the prospects for recovery.

The extraordinary recent advances in basic neuroscience research have provided significant new opportunities for understanding the linkages between the brain and behavior and for incorporating this knowledge into studies of human health. Simultaneously, behavioral and social science research is increasingly interdisciplinary. The variables that affect health and illness may occur at the molecular, cellular, organ system, behavioral and psychological, and social and environmental levels.[3] Recognizing these interactions often requires a broad understanding of the connections between the behavioral sciences, findings from basic biomedical laboratories (especially in pharmacology and biochemistry), and the practice of medicine and public health.

After weighing these factors and reviewing the extent to which graduate education in various behavioral science fields is supported by the National Institutes of Health (NIH), we defined the target workforce for our study as Ph.D.s trained in anthropology, demography, the nonclinical fields of psychology, sociology, and the speech and hearing sciences (see Appendix E). Those who graduate from universities in the U.S. with Ph.D.s in these fields and seek careers in science and engineering in this country are considered part of the behavioral and social science workforce until they retire, die, or leave science and engineering for another field of work.

An analysis of Ph.D.s in these fields will unavoid-

[1] National Research Council. *Biomedical and Behavioral Research Scientists: Their Training and Supply. Volume 1: Findings.* Washington, D.C.: National Academy Press, 1989.

[2] National Research Council. *Meeting the Nation's Needs for Biomedical and Behavioral Scientists.* Washington, D.C.: National Academy Press, 1994.

[3] Anderson, Norman B. "Levels of Analysis in Health Science: A Framework for Integrating Sociobehavioral and Biomedical Research." *Annals of the New York Academy of Sciences* 840 (May 1998): 563-76.

ably include investigators who do not pursue health-related research and exclude others from related fields who may be actively involved in such studies. Economists, for example, were not included in our analysis, even though studies of the economics of health and medicine make major contributions to health-related research. Because less than 2 percent of the nation's economists focus on health economics,[4] including this field in our analysis would overestimate the size of the workforce. Nonetheless, the definition of the behavioral and social science workforce described above can provide a general estimate of the number of investigators in this field and an indication of the major trends affecting the workforce, such as changes in size, age, and composition.

A PORTRAIT OF THE WORKFORCE

As in the basic biomedical sciences, the behavioral and social science workforce has more than doubled since 1975, from just over 25,800 Ph.D.s to 57,800 in 1997 (see Figure 3-1). In contrast to the steady growth of the basic biomedical workforce during that period, most of the increase in the behavioral and social sciences occurred between 1975 and 1989, when the size of the workforce climbed from 25,802 to 48,844 Ph.D.s. Growth slowed markedly thereafter, and by 1995 the workforce totaled 52,324 Ph.D.s. By 1997 the number of behavioral and social scientists had jumped again, to 57,843.

This recent growth, however, should be interpreted with caution. A change in the survey methodology in 1993 may have affected subsequent estimates of workforce size by classifying individuals by occupation (e.g., scientist, professor, manager), rather than by scientific field. In addition, part of this reported workforce growth stems from a change in the analysis of survey responses by the National Opinion Research Center when it took over the management of the Survey of Doctorate Recipients in 1997.

Since 1975 the representation of women and minorities in the behavioral and social science workforce has grown significantly (see Figure 3-2). In the mid-1970s, 20.5 percent of the behavioral science workforce were women and 2.5 percent were minorities. Since then, as increasing numbers of women and minorities have earned Ph.D.s in these fields, their representation in the workforce has steadily risen. By 1997, 41.9 percent of behavioral and social scientists were women and 6.9 percent were minorities.

In the absence of a rapid increase of new Ph.D.s, as seen in the basic biomedical sciences, the median age of the behavioral and social science workforce has grown over the last decade, rising from 44.4 in 1987 to

[4] Sikes, Violet. American Economic Association. Personal communication, October 1999.

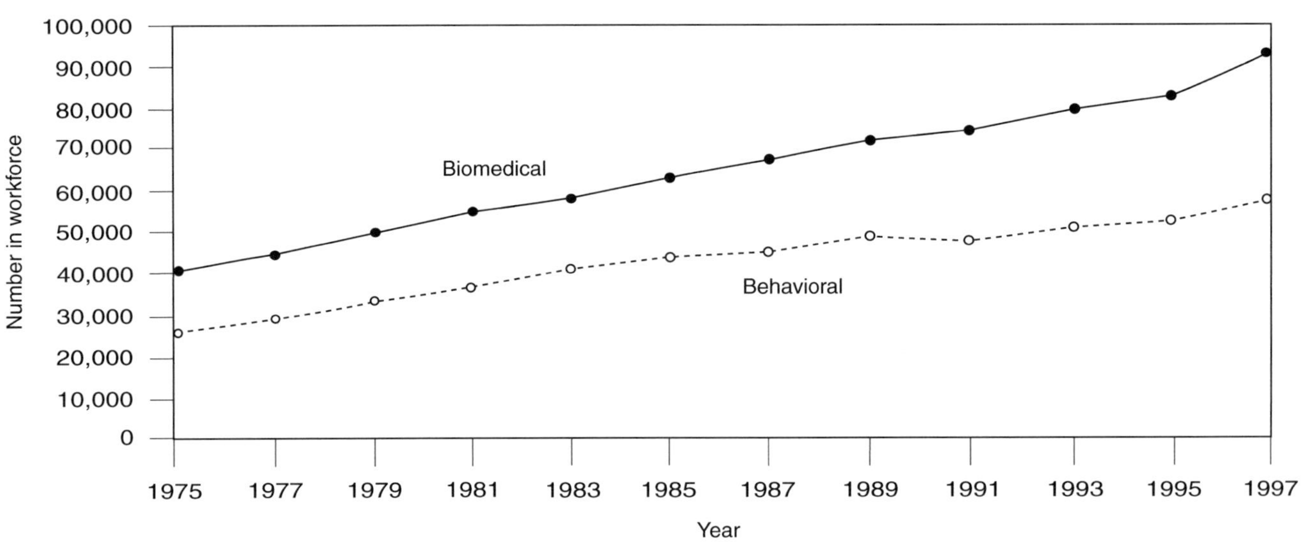

FIGURE 3-1 Growth in the behavioral and social science workforce and the basic biomedical workforce. SOURCE: Data are from the Survey of Doctorate Recipients (see Tables G-4 and G-5).

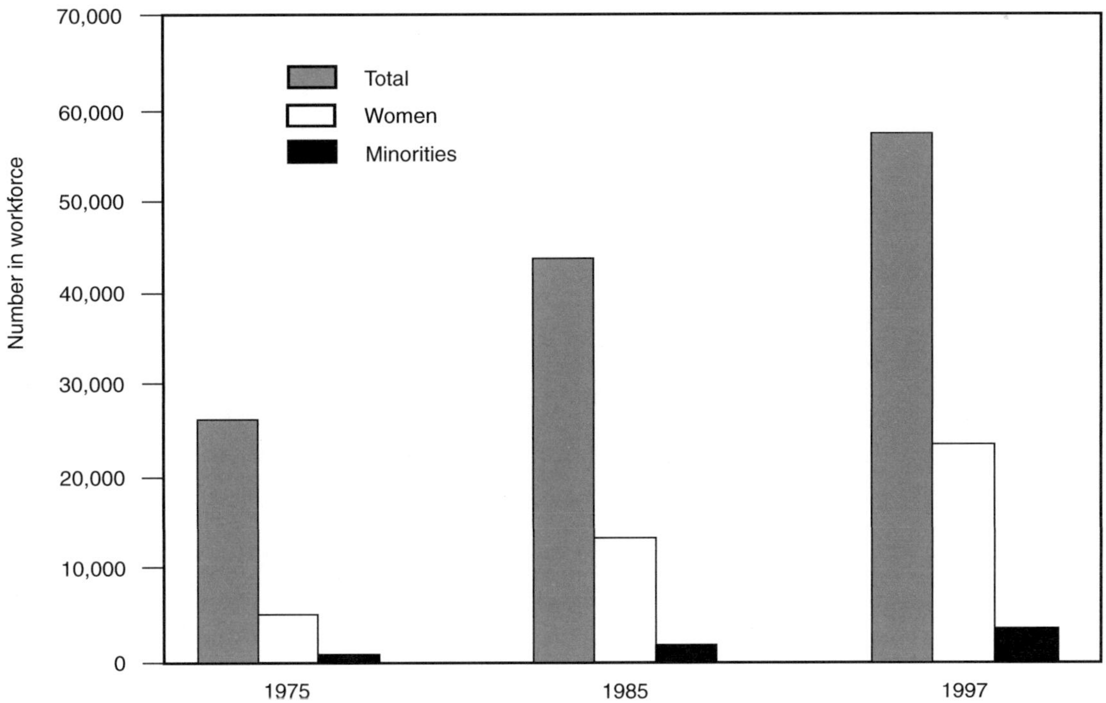

FIGURE 3-2 Trends in the composition of the behavioral and social science workforce. SOURCE: Data are from the Survey of Doctorate Recipients (see Table G-5).

49.8 in 1997.[5] A demographic analysis of the workforce (described in Appendix D) estimates that the median age of the behavioral and social sciences workforce likely will increase by another two and one-half years by 2005 to 52.4 years. In contrast, the median age of the biomedical workforce is expected to grow less than a year during that period to 46.2.

Unless there is a major departure from current trends in Ph.D. production and retirement, the behavioral and social science workforce is projected to continue growing at a rate of more than 1 percent annually for the next several years. By 2005 this workforce is expected to number nearly 60,000 and include almost equal numbers of men and women.

TRENDS IN THE EDUCATION OF BEHAVIORAL AND SOCIAL SCIENTISTS

Many of the changes in the behavioral and social science workforce reflect trends in doctoral education over the past 25 years. Increasing numbers of women, underrepresented minorities, and noncitizens have obtained doctoral degrees in the behavioral and social sciences, just as in the basic biomedical sciences. In addition, the time spent earning a Ph.D. in the behavioral and social sciences has grown. Postdoctoral study is not as customary for behavioral and social science Ph.D.s as for those in biomedical fields but has been slowly increasing.

In many other regards, doctoral education in the behavioral and social sciences differs markedly from that in the basic biomedical sciences. Unlike the biomedical fields, in which steadily increasing numbers of Ph.D.s have been awarded since the mid-1970s, the number of advanced degrees earned in the behavioral and social sciences has been rising only since the start of the 1990s, reversing a modest but extended decline that began in the late 1970s and continued throughout the 1980s (see Figure 3-3).

Another area of difference between the two fields is the number of degrees awarded to men (see Figure 3-4). Since peaking at 1,949 in 1976, the number of men receiving Ph.D.s in the behavioral and social sciences has dropped considerably. Men earned less than 40 percent (1,012) of the 2,591 behavioral and social sci-

[5] Unpublished tabulation from the Survey of Doctorate Recipients; available from the archives of the Academies.

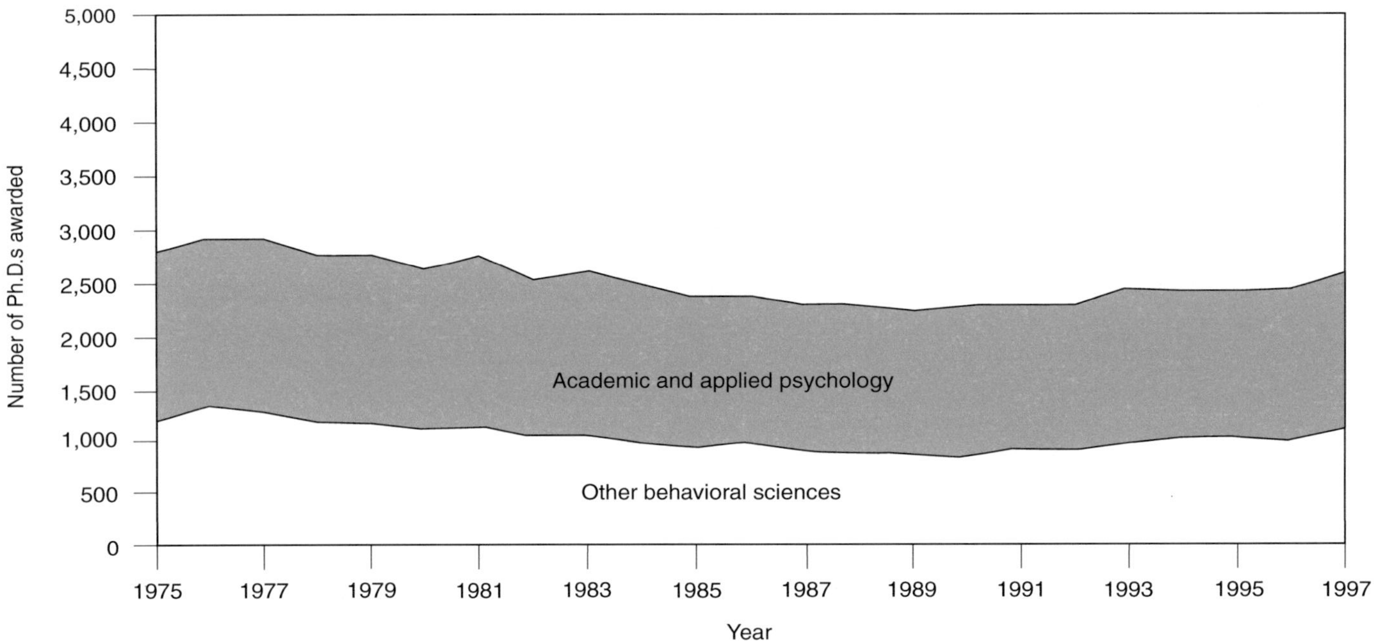

FIGURE 3-3 Ph.D.s awarded in the behavioral and social sciences in the United States. SOURCE: Data are from the Survey of Earned Doctorates (see Table G-2).

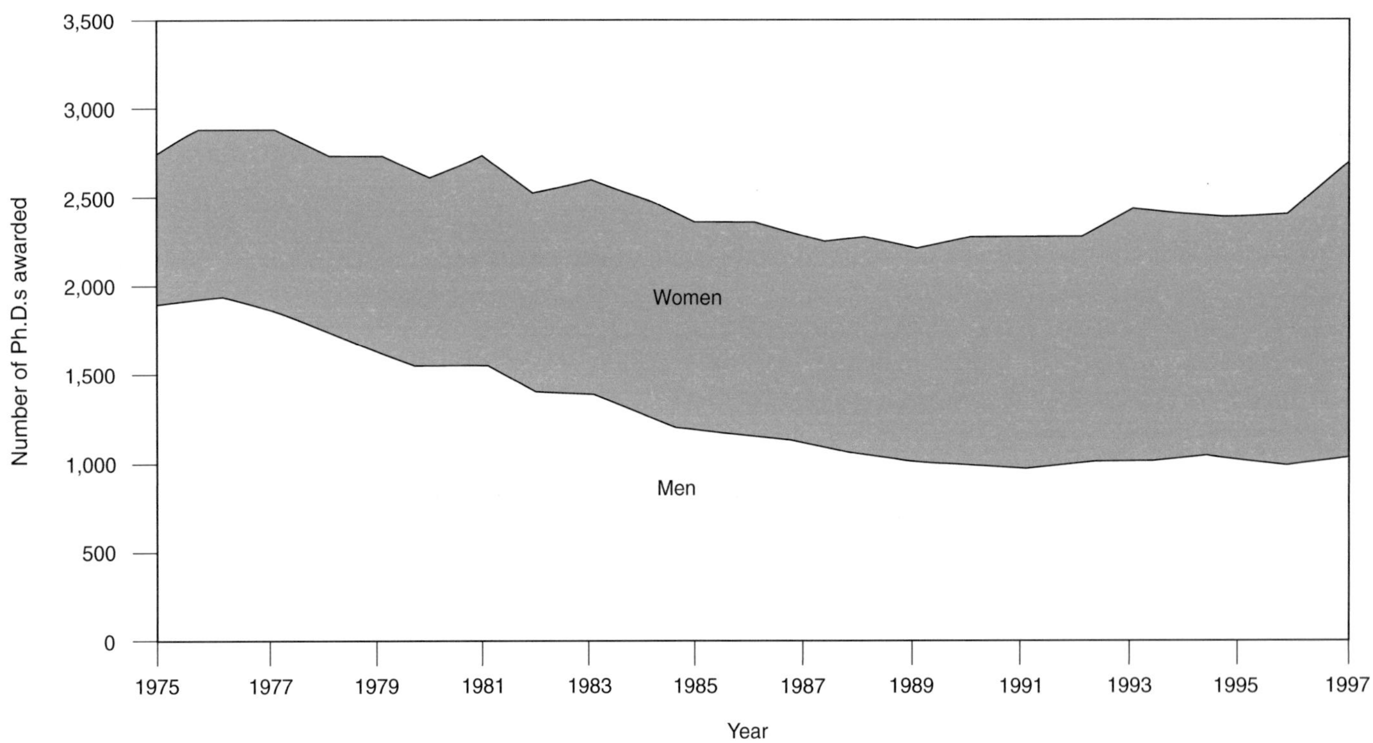

FIGURE 3-4 Ph.D.s awarded in the behavioral and social sciences in the United States by gender. SOURCE: Data are from the Survey of Earned Doctorates (see Table G-2).

ence Ph.D.s granted in 1997. As a result, the growth in behavioral and social science Ph.D.s granted in the 1990s is due almost entirely to the increasing numbers of women earning doctoral degrees in these fields. In 1975 women earned just under a third (895) of the Ph.D.s awarded in the behavioral and social sciences; since then their numbers have steadily grown, reaching 1,558 in 1997.

The behavioral and social sciences also differ from the biomedical fields in the fraction of Ph.D.s awarded to underrepresented minorities. Though minorities have earned increasing numbers and percentages of advanced degrees in both fields, they have always been better represented in the behavioral and social sciences. In 1975 underrepresented minorities earned 114 doctoral degrees in the behavioral and social sciences (4.1 percent of the degrees awarded that year); by 1997 that number had grown to 219 (8.5 percent). In contrast, underrepresented minorities earned 4.7 percent of Ph.D.s awarded in the basic biomedical sciences in 1997.

The fraction of behavioral and social science Ph.D.s awarded to noncitizens has also increased, though not as steadily as, and much less dramatically than, in the basic biomedical sciences. The percentage of doctoral degrees in the behavioral and social sciences awarded to individuals holding temporary visas increased from 6.8 percent in 1975 to 12.9 percent in 1993. The percentage of degrees earned by temporary-visa holders decreased to 9.8 percent in 1997.

Along with these other changes, the number of years spent earning a Ph.D. in the behavioral and social sciences increased sharply from the mid-1970s to the late 1980s. Although time to degree has declined slightly since then, doctoral recipients in 1997 received their degrees 8.8 years after beginning graduate study, in contrast to the six and one-quarter years typical for those graduating in 1975 (median time to degree as measured from entry into post-baccalaureate study). As a result, the median age of new Ph.D.s in the behavioral and social sciences today is 33.4, three years older than those who graduated in the mid-1970s.

Time to degree and the median age of new Ph.D.s have always been greater in the behavioral and social sciences than in the biomedical disciplines, but the disparity between the two fields has grown over the last two decades. The basic biomedical Ph.D.s awarded their degrees in 1997 completed their graduate studies in 7.8 years, at a median age of 30.9.

Of course, a career in the basic biomedical sciences today almost invariably requires a postdoctoral fellowship, which extends the time spent in training. Though on the increase, postdoctoral study is not the norm for most behavioral and social science Ph.D.s; 18.8 percent of new Ph.D.s in the behavioral and social sciences in 1997 reported plans for postdoctoral study, up from 12.5 percent in 1975. In contrast, nearly two-thirds of 1997 Ph.D.s in the basic biomedical sciences expected to pursue postdoctoral study.

TRENDS IN EMPLOYMENT

Though behavioral and social science Ph.D.s are most often employed in academia today, as was the case in the past, increasing numbers are pursuing professional opportunities in other arenas. For the purposes of this analysis, those holding postdoctoral appointments are considered to be in the workforce. As indicated in Figure 3-5, the number of behavioral and social scientists who work in industry or are self-employed has climbed from 2,111 (8.2 percent of the workforce) in 1975 to 11,779 (20.4 percent of the workforce) today. Government employment has also increased, though at a somewhat slower pace. Today, 5,192 behavioral and social science Ph.D.s, or 9 percent of the workforce, are employed in government, up from 1,793 in 1975. During the same period, the number of behavioral and social science Ph.D.s working in academia grew from 18,668 to 34,850. Because positions in academia did not increase as fast as in other sectors, the fraction of the behavioral and social science workforce working in academia declined from 72.4 percent in 1975 to 60.2 percent in 1997.

More recently, however, the number of new positions available in industry appears to be leveling off, and greater numbers of Ph.D.s are once more finding employment in academia. Unlike the 1970s, however, when nearly all academic hiring was for faculty positions, the jobs available in academia today are more evenly split between faculty and nonfaculty appointments (see Figure 3-6). Almost 21 percent of behavioral and social science Ph.D.s employed in academia in 1997 held postdoctoral or "other academic" appointments (i.e., nonfaculty positions as research associates or instructors). Furthermore, faculty appointments today are somewhat less likely to offer tenure. In 1975, 96.1 percent of behavioral and social science faculty were tenured or held tenure-track appointments; the same was true for 88.5 percent of faculty in 1997.

Since the early 1990s, when many new psychology

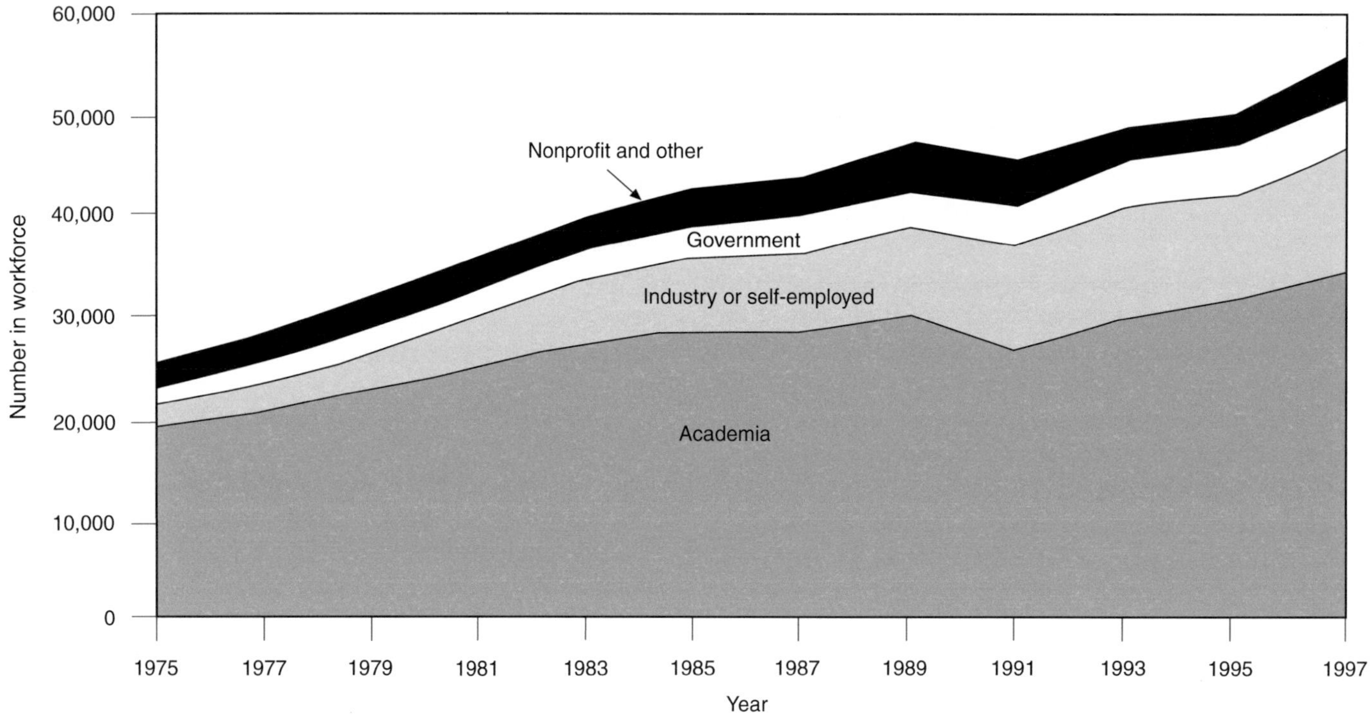

FIGURE 3-5 Employment of behavioral and social scientists by sector. SOURCE: Data are from the Survey of Doctorate Recipients (see Table G-5).

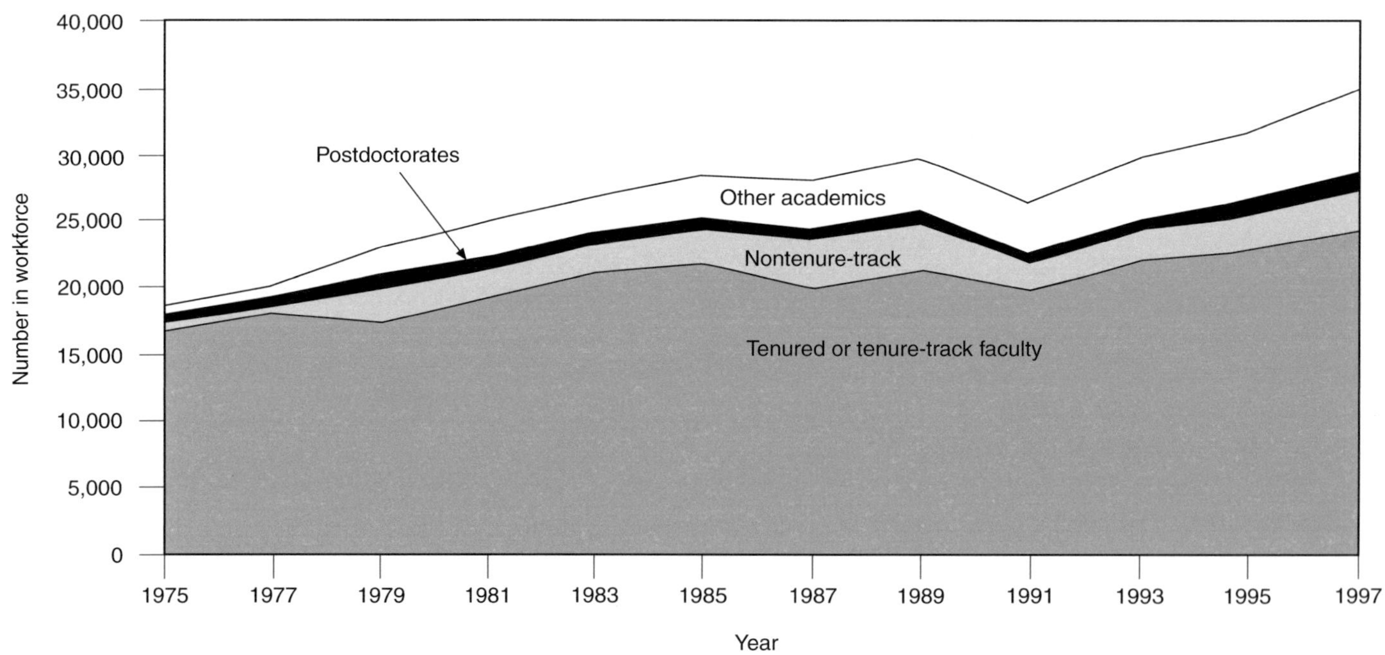

FIGURE 3-6 Employment of behavioral and social scientists in academia. SOURCE: Data are from the Survey of Doctorate Recipients (see Table G-5).

Ph.D.s reported difficulties finding a position, the job market has improved. In 1993 and 1995 only 25 percent of the recent doctoral recipients from the nonclinical specialties of psychology described the job market as "good" or "excellent."[6] By 1997 more than 40 percent of new Ph.D.s rated the job market as "good" or better. In addition, departments of psychology have begun to offer faculty appointments to increasing numbers of new Ph.D.s.[7] For the 1998-1999 academic year, U.S. graduate departments of psychology hired 186 new faculty members trained in nonclinical fields, an increase of almost 45 percent over the previous year.

While encouraging, these improvements in the job market do not necessarily mean that Ph.D. production in the behavioral and social sciences should increase. If the behavioral science workforce were to grow at a rate comparable to that projected for the U.S. workforce as a whole until 2005, the number of new Ph.D.s necessary each year would be slightly less than current levels of Ph.D. production (see Appendix D). Despite the recent upturn in hiring, fewer opportunities for new Ph.D.s to obtain faculty positions are available than a decade ago, when departments of psychology appointed 255 recent doctoral recipients from nonclinical specialties to their faculties.

THE CHANGING ROLE OF THE NATIONAL RESEARCH SERVICE AWARD PROGRAM

In general, the National Research Service Award (NRSA) program plays a smaller role in research training in the behavioral and social sciences than in the basic biomedical fields. Just under 10 percent of U.S. citizens and permanent residents earning behavioral and social science Ph.D.s in 1995 received NRSA funding at some point during their predoctoral study, compared to nearly 35 percent in the basic biomedical sciences.[8] In part, this is because a great deal of behavioral and social research training is unrelated to health and is supported by the National Science Foundation rather than the NIH. Funding from NRSA training grants and fellowships is relatively more common for the behavioral and social sciences fields with strong ties to health research. Nearly 30 percent of the 85 eligible Ph.D.s in physiological psychology in 1995 were supported by NRSA funding during their predoctoral studies; the same was true for nearly 25 percent of the 134 eligible degree recipients in developmental and child psychology and more than 70 percent of the seven eligible Ph.D.s in demography.[9]

The most recent assessment of the career outcomes of NRSA predoctoral trainees and fellows in the behavioral and social sciences, conducted in the late 1990s, did not yield results that were as clear-cut as a similar evaluation of NRSA training in the basic biomedical sciences described in Chapter 2. NRSA trainees and fellows, particularly those who received support at the start of graduate school, completed their Ph.D.s faster than other students in the behavioral and social sciences.[10] Yet in subsequent employment and research, no clear differences could be detected between NRSA recipients and other Ph.D.s in these fields. These findings, however, should be interpreted with caution. The information on career outcomes for this evaluation was obtained from sample surveys, and the fraction of NRSA recipients in the behavioral sciences is much smaller than in the biomedical sciences. As a result, the capacity to detect meaningful differences in the career outcomes of behavioral scientists was limited.

Federal support for graduate education in the behavioral and social sciences has followed the same pattern seen in the basic biomedical sciences: declining numbers of students supported by training grants and fellowships, and a steady increase in students working as research assistants. As illustrated in Figure 3-7, nearly four times as many students received their primary support from NIH (or other DHHS) traineeships and fellowships in 1975 as from research grants. Yet today, graduate students employed as research assistants under federal grants outnumber those supported by training grants or fellowships by more than two to one.

A similar though less pronounced reversal has occurred in the federal funding of postdoctoral positions

[6] Unpublished tabulation from the American Psychological Association, Doctorate Employment Survey; available from the archives of the Academies.

[7] Unpublished tabulation from the American Psychological Association, Faculty Salary Survey; available from the archives of the Academies.

[8] Unpublished tabulation from the Survey of Earned Doctorates and NIH Trainee and Fellow File; available from the archives of the Academies.

[9] Ibid.

[10] Pion, Georgine M. Office of Extramural Research, National Institutes of Health. *The Early Career Progress of NRSA Predoctoral Trainees and Fellows.* Bethesda, Md.: NIH, 2000.

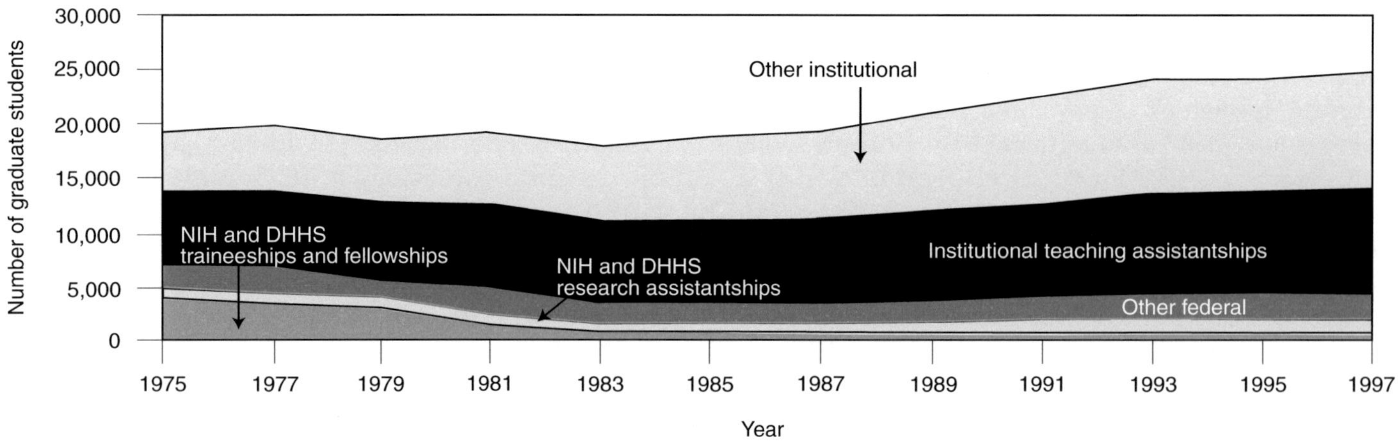

FIGURE 3-7 Trends in graduate students' primary source of support in the behavioral and social sciences. Includes all students at doctorate-granting universities, whether candidates for master's or doctoral degrees, and all subfields of psychology. SOURCE: Data are from the Survey of Graduate Students and Postdoctorates in Science and Engineering (see Table G-8).

in the behavioral and social sciences. In 1975, the majority (53.4 percent) of federally funded postdoctorates in the behavioral and social sciences were supported through training grants or fellowships.[11] By 1997, the majority (52.8 percent) were employed on research grants; the share of those with funding from training grants and fellowships had declined to 47.2 percent.

The NIH's efforts to shift research training in the behavioral and social sciences from the predoctoral to the postdoctoral level in the late 1970s and 1980s (described in Chapter 1) account for much of the reduction in training grant and fellowship support for graduate students in these fields. The reason for the concurrent rise in graduate research assistantships is less clear, but may result from a combination of factors. The rising number of graduate research assistants is likely influenced by the funding practices of the NIH, which provides almost $9,000 more to research assistants and their institutions than to its NRSA trainees or fellows, mostly in the form of indirect cost payments to universities (see Table 2-1). In addition, the reliance on research assistantships has grown in conjunction with the number of graduate students in this country on temporary visas, who are not eligible for NRSA awards. Finally, though the size of the NRSA program has been monitored closely to ensure that the number of trainees and fellows participating in its programs corresponded to national needs, no similar federal effort has been undertaken to ensure an adequate supply of technically prepared support staff in research, nor is there a system for regulating the number of research assistantships. As a result, Massy and Goldman concluded in their 1995 analysis of science and engineering Ph.D. production that the size of doctoral programs is driven largely by departmental needs for research and teaching assistants, rather than by the labor market for Ph.D.s.[12] Unlike biomedical and clinical research training, which tends to be widely distributed among the NIH institutes, relatively few institutes are responsible for the bulk of the agency's behavioral research training. The National Institute of Mental Health supports the majority of NRSA trainees and fellows in the behavioral and social sciences (55.3 percent in 1997), followed by the National Institute of Child Health and Human Development (13.1 percent), the National Institute on Aging (11.7 percent), the National Institute on Drug Abuse (5.1 percent), and the National Institute on Alcohol Abuse and Alcoholism (4.1 percent).[13]

[11] Unpublished tabulation from the Survey of Graduate Students and Postdoctorates in Science and Engineering; available from the archives of the Academies.

[12] Massy, William F., and Charles A. Goldman. *The Production and Utilization of Science and Engineering Doctorates in the United States.* Stanford Institute for Higher Education Research Discussion Paper. Stanford, Calif.: 1995.

[13] Unpublished tabulation from the Survey of Earned Doctorates and NIH Trainee and Fellow File; available from the archives of the Academies.

For graduate students participating in NRSA programs today, research training in behavioral and social science fields often focuses on a single discipline, such as psychology. In contrast to research training in basic biomedical sciences, where the NIH has mandated that most training grants be multidisciplinary, neither the NIMH nor other institutes active in behavioral research training have required multidisciplinary or interdisciplinary research training.

The predoctoral fellowships offered by the National Institute of Mental Health, National Institute on Drug Abuse, and National Institute on Alcohol Abuse and Alcoholism for M.D.-Ph.D. training might be expected to provide opportunities for interdisciplinary training in behavior and medicine. Yet these fellowships are generally limited to those enrolled in existing M.D.-Ph.D. programs,[14] which typically emphasize basic biomedical training. Consequently, almost all fellows to date have graduated with a Ph.D. in a biomedical discipline, rather than a degree in one of the behavioral or social sciences.[15]

Recently, however, several NIH institutes and offices have advocated interdisciplinary research training in the behavioral and social sciences. In reports issued in 1997 and 1998, the NIH-wide Office of Behavioral and Social Science Research and the National Heart, Lung, and Blood Institute recommended more interdisciplinary behavioral research training to foster enhanced communication and collaboration between behavioral, biomedical, and clinical researchers and to encourage such investigators to "become familiar with each others' methods and procedures."[16-17] In early 1999 the National Institute of Mental Health, the National Institute on Aging, the National Institute of Nursing Research, and the NIH Office of Behavioral and Social Science Research asked the Institute of Medicine to study approaches to interdisciplinary research training in the brain, behavioral, and clinical sciences and to develop recommendations for its expansion; that study is now underway.[18]

IMPLICATIONS AND RECOMMENDATIONS

At present, the overall size of the behavioral and social science workforce is sufficient to fill existing national needs, and current levels of research training appear to be adequate to maintain that supply. The extent to which these findings apply to the portion of the behavioral and social science workforce that conducts health research is less clear. No evidence suggests that circumstances differ for those conducting health-related research, but future analyses of this workforce will undoubtedly benefit from a better understanding of the number of behavioral and social science Ph.D.s engaged in health-related research, their training, and career patterns.

In reports issued in 1997 and 1998, the NIH-wide Office of Behavioral and Social Science Research and the National Heart, Lung, and Blood Institute recommended that the agency's research training programs take a more interdisciplinary approach to training in the behavioral and social sciences. Given the extraordinary opportunities for applying advances in the brain sciences and imaging technology to behavioral research and the growing appreciation of the role that behavior plays in clinical medicine and public health today, we strongly support such recommendations. An interdisciplinary approach to research training will undoubtedly benefit young investigators and strengthen behavioral and social sciences research overall. Broader training will provide behavioral and social science investigators with the capacity to work in a greater variety of employment settings and apply their training to a wider range of research problems, including those that require an understanding of neuroscience (and related fields such as pharmacology and biochemistry), clinical medicine, and public health.

Transforming research training in the behavioral and social sciences into a more interdisciplinary activity is likely to be a major undertaking that will require a con-

[14] "Individual Predoctoral National Research Service Awards for M.D.-Ph.D. Fellowships." *NIH Guide for Grants and Contracts*, 20 April 1999. Available: http://grants.nih.gov/grants/guide/index.html.

[15] Unpublished tabulation from the Survey of Earned Doctorates and NIH Trainee and Fellow File; available from the archives of the Academies.

[16] National Institutes of Health. National Heart, Lung, and Blood Institute. *Report of the Task Force on Behavioral Research in Cardiovascular, Lung, and Blood Health and Disease*. Bethesda, Md.: NIH, 1998.

[17] National Institutes of Health. Office of Behavioral and Social Sciences Research. *A Strategic Plan for the Office of Behavioral and Social Sciences Research at the National Institutes of Health*. Bethesda, Md.: NIH, 1997.

[18] National Academies. Current Project System. "Building Bridges in the Brain, Behavioral, and Clinical Sciences." Online. Available: http://www4.nas.edu/cp.nsf. Accessed 25 August 1999.

certed effort by the NIH and changes in several facets of its research training programs. Rather than suggest a single approach, we recommend that the agency consider the following:

- Gradually shift the focus of its predoctoral programs from single discipline to interdisciplinary training.
- Increase the opportunities for postdoctoral training through interdisciplinary training grants.
- Involve more NIH institutes in behavioral and social science research training, either independently or in joint activities with the institutes that already support the bulk of this training.
- Monitor more closely the implementation of the 1997 policy change for M.D.-Ph.D. programs to ensure that more students are provided opportunities to pursue studies in the behavioral and social sciences related to medicine.

Whatever strategies the NIH chooses, NRSA training mechanisms provide an obvious opportunity for interdisciplinary research training and warrant expansion. Research assistantships, which generally require recipients to focus on a specific research question, are less likely to provide students and postdoctorates with a broad understanding of the interdisciplinary connections between fields. It is unlikely, however, that the NIH could readily return to the pattern of federal research training support that existed in the mid-1970s when the NRSA program was initiated and more than 80 percent of graduate students in the behavioral sciences with NIH or other DHHS support received funding through training grants or fellowships. Instead, the committee believes that the agency should strive for a middle ground: gradually expanding the NRSA program until it accounts for at least 50 percent of the agency's funding for graduate students in the behavioral and social sciences and correspondingly limiting research assistantships and other modes of graduate student support to ensure that overall Ph.D. production does not increase. At the postdoctoral level, the NIH should also seek to provide advanced research training to a greater number of recent Ph.D.s through NRSA training grants and fellowships, rather than postdoctoral appointments on research grants.

Coordinating reciprocal increases in the NRSA program and reductions in other funding for graduate student support will undoubtedly require the NIH to consolidate its oversight of research training and training-related activities. Such a change in NIH policies and procedures will also have implications for the conduct of research and the ways in which universities administer federal research training funds and will require careful monitoring by the NIH. These and related issues are discussed in greater detail in Chapter 5.

Finally, the NIH should also continue to focus attention on the training of underrepresented minorities in the behavioral and social sciences. The numbers of minority students earning Ph.D.s in the behavioral and social sciences have steadily increased over the last 25 years, but these trends will need further monitoring to ensure that the workforce better reflects the nation's increasing diversity and that the workforce is prepared to address the nation's changing health needs.

Recommendation 3-1. The NIH and the National Science Foundation should take steps to improve data on the behavioral and social sciences workforce, so that those conducting health-related research can be specifically identified in national surveys of the scientific workforce.

> Unlike the basic biomedical science workforce, which focuses almost exclusively on health-related research, Ph.D.s trained in the behavioral and social sciences pursue a broader research agenda, much of which is unrelated to health and medicine. At present, investigators trained in health-related research cannot be identified or tracked, which limits any analysis of the nation's needs.

Recommendation 3-2. There should be no growth in the aggregate number of Ph.D.s awarded annually in the behavioral and social sciences.

> Given the current employment opportunities for behavioral and social scientists and the continuing growth forecast in the workforce, the present number of approximately 2,600 new behavioral and social science Ph.D.s per year is sufficient to fulfill anticipated national needs in the near future (until at least 2005).

Recommendation 3-3. The NIH should increase its emphasis on interdisciplinary research training in the behavioral and social sciences.

> Research training in the behavioral and social sciences related to health should be expanded beyond traditional disciplinary boundaries and provide opportunities for participating students and fellows to

integrate their knowledge of the behavioral and social sciences with advances in the brain sciences (and related fields such as brain imaging, biochemistry, and pharmacology), public health, and medicine.

Transforming research training in the behavioral and social sciences into a more interdisciplinary activity is likely to require a concerted effort by the NIH and changes in several facets of its research training programs. Rather than recommend a single approach, we suggest that the agency consider the following options for achieving this goal:

- Gradually shift the focus of its predoctoral programs from single-discipline to interdisciplinary training.
- Increase the opportunities for postdoctoral training through interdisciplinary training grants.
- Involve more NIH institutes in behavioral and social science research training, either independently or in joint activities with the institutes that already support the bulk of this training.
- Monitor more closely the implementation of the 1997 policy change for M.D.-Ph.D. programs, to ensure that more students are provided opportunities to pursue studies in the behavioral and social sciences related to medicine.

Recommendation 3-4. Support for NRSA training grants and fellowships at the predoctoral and postdoctorals level should be gradually increased. At the predoctoral level, the NIH should seek to provide at least 50 percent of its research training support through training grants and fellowships.

The committee believes that training grants and fellowships are more conducive to interdisciplinary research training and career development than are research assistantships and is concerned by the relative shift away from NRSA training mechanisms toward research assistantships to support students and postdoctorates in the biomedical and behavioral sciences that has occurred since 1975. Therefore, we recommend a gradual expansion in the numbers of students and postdoctorates supported by NRSA training grants and fellowships, but only if accompanied by a change in the pattern of NIH support: more training funded via NRSA mechanisms and less training supported by research grants.

NIH should carefully monitor the effects of this change on the conduct of research and research training and should consider options to assist graduate departments in restricting the expansion of Ph.D. programs, including (1) encouraging universities to provide all entering graduate students with some form of financial support, such as a traineeship, that would allow them an opportunity for broad multidisciplinary education, (2) requiring graduate students to pass qualifying exams before working as research assistants on federally funded projects, and (3) limiting the number of years graduate students and postdoctorates may be employed in temporary appointments with federal funds.

Recommendation 3-5. The NIH should continue its efforts to identify and support programs that encourage and prepare underrepresented minority students for careers in behavioral and social science research.

Although the number of underrepresented minority men and women earning Ph.D.s in the behavioral and social sciences has increased substantially in recent years, the NIH should take steps to ensure that these trends continue and accelerate.

4

Clinical Scientists

IDENTIFYING THE WORKFORCE

Of the three groups that make up the health research workforce, clinical investigators are the most difficult to identify and track. In part, this is a result of the increasing diversity of this sector of the research workforce, which was once dominated by physicians but now includes increasing numbers of Ph.D.s. Assessment of this workforce is also complicated by a lack of information about the research training and career paths of physicians and other health care professionals, who necessarily play a major role in the field of clinical research.

The dearth of information about such health care doctorates as physicians, dentists, and other doctoral-level professionals without Ph.D.s is a longstanding problem, identified by the first NRC committee to examine the needs for biomedical and behavioral researchers in 1975[1] and regularly cited as an obstacle by subsequent committees.[2,3] Only in the last few years has more detailed information become available, after the National Institutes of Health (NIH) adopted a definition of clinical research and began collecting information about its grants and the investigators who receive them. In keeping with its new policy, implemented in 1996, the NIH classifies studies as clinical research when they fall into one of three categories: (1) patient-oriented research, including clinical trials, the development of new technologies, studies of therapeutic interventions, and the mechanisms of human disease, (2) epidemiological and behavioral studies, or (3) outcomes and health services research.[4] Although the Agency for Healthcare Research and Quality (AHRQ) does not categorize the research it funds in the same fashion, the studies it supports generally fall within the parameters for clinical research established by the NIH.

In fiscal year 1997, almost 23 percent of the approximately 12,000 new and competing grants awarded by the NIH were for clinical research projects.[5] Because the grant portfolio of the AHRQ is much smaller, combining it with that of the NIH does not increase significantly the percentage of clinical research projects supported by the two agencies (see Table 4-1). The majority of principal investigators for clinical research projects supported by NIH and AHRQ held Ph.D.s (1,449), rather than M.D.s or M.D.-Ph.D.s (1,061).

As indicated in Table 4-1, a much larger fraction of researchers with M.D.s than with Ph.D.s were involved in clinical research. More than any other group of investigators receiving grants from the NIH and AHRQ in 1997, M.D.s were most likely to conduct clinical research (36.3 percent). At 29.6 percent, "other" degree holders ranked next in conducting clinical research

[1] National Research Council. *Personnel Needs and Training for Biomedical and Behavioral Research.* Washington, D.C.: National Academy of Sciences, 1975.

[2] National Research Council. *Personnel Needs and Training for Biomedical and Behavioral Research.* Washington, D.C.: National Academy of Sciences, 1976.

[3] National Research Council. *Biomedical and Behavioral Research Scientists: Their Training and Supply. Volume 1: Findings.* Washington, D.C.: National Academy Press, 1989.

[4] National Institutes of Health. Director's Panel on Clinical Research. *Report to the Advisory Committee to the NIH Director.* Bethesda, Md.: NIH, 1997.

[5] Unpublished tabulation from the NIH CRISP and IMPAC systems; on file in the archives of the Academies.

TABLE 4-1 NIH and AHRQ Competing Awards by Type of Research and Degree of Investigator, Fiscal Year 1997

	M.D.		M.D.-Ph.D.		Ph.D.		Other[a]		Total	
Type of Research	No.	Percent	No.	Percent	No.	Percent	No.	Percent	No.	Percent
Clinical	959	36.3	102	21.3	1,449	18.0	257	29.6	2,767	23.0
Nonclinical	1,682	63.7	376	78.7	6,593	82.0	611	70.4	9,262	77.0
Total	2,641	100.0	478	100.0	8,042	100.0	868	100.0	12,029	100.0

NOTE: NIH data exclude training grants and predoctoral fellowships. AHRQ data exclude training grants, predoctoral fellowships, innovation awards, and conference grants.

[a] This category includes dentists and veterinarians, as well as investigators for whom no degree information was available.

SOURCES: Data are from the NIH CRISP and IMPAC systems and the *AHCPR State List of Active Grants*.

(perhaps reflecting the fact that dentists are included in this group), followed by M.D.-Ph.D.s (21.3 percent). As a group, Ph.D.s were least likely to conduct clinical research: only 18 percent did so.

DEFINING CLINICAL RESEARCH AND THE CLINICAL RESEARCH WORKFORCE

Previous NRC analyses of clinical research have generally assumed that Ph.D.s conducting clinical research were trained in the health science disciplines listed in Appendix E, including fields such as environmental health, epidemiology, health services, nursing, and pharmacy. Yet the data on federally funded clinical research collected over the last few years reveal a workforce that is much more complex than previously recognized. According to this new information, the pool of investigators conducting clinical research supported by the NIH and AHRQ includes many who were trained in the behavioral and social sciences and, to a lesser extent, the basic biomedical sciences.

Among those whose fields of study could be identified, more Ph.D.s conducting clinical research received their degrees in clinical psychology (13.4 percent) than in any other discipline. Other fields producing large numbers of clinical investigators (listed in Table 4-2) included such traditional disciplines as epidemiology and nursing, as well as those less commonly associated with clinical research, including sociology, biochemistry, and physiology.

By adopting a definition of clinical research that encompasses behavioral and social science studies, the

TABLE 4-2 Ph.D.s Receiving NIH Awards for Clinical Research, by Field of Degree, 1998

Field of degree	Number	Percent
Clinical psychology	142	13.4
Experimental psychology	60	5.7
Sociology	52	4.9
Epidemiology	42	4.0
Nursing	40	3.8
Biochemistry	36	3.4
Psychology, general	36	3.4
Social psychology	35	3.3
Developmental and child psychology	31	2.9
Physiology	26	2.5
Genetics (human and animal)	23	2.2
Molecular biology	23	2.2
Speech-language pathology and audiology	23	2.2
Physiological psychology/psychobiology	21	2.0
Bioengineering and biomedical engineering	21	2.0
Anthropology	19	1.8
Other Fields	437	41.4
Total identified	1,056	100.0
Unknown fields	347	
Total	1,403	

SOURCES: Principal investigators were identified from the NIH CRISP and IMPAC Systems and matched against data from the Survey of Earned Doctorates to determine the fields in which they earned their doctoral degrees.

NIH has recognized the links and inevitable overlap between the two fields. The committee applauds this development in NIH policy and hopes that it will encourage more cross-disciplinary research on the behavioral and social factors so critical to the nation's health. However, this definition of clinical research creates some complications for evaluating the clinical research workforce.

Because there is no simple way, for example, to predict which clinical psychology Ph.D.s will pursue careers in research and which will focus on clinical practice or to distinguish biochemists and sociologists in clinical research from those pursuing laboratory or other types of research (unless they have received funding from the NIH since 1996), we did not include these investigators in our assessments of the size and characteristics of the clinical research workforce, opting instead to rely on the traditional taxonomy of health science Ph.D.s (see Appendix E). Nonetheless, it is important to keep in mind that investigators from fields other than the health sciences play a significant role in clinical research. Future studies of this workforce should consider approaches that better account for these Ph.D.s, especially clinical psychologists, who were not included in our analysis of the behavioral and social science workforce.

GAUGING THE SIZE AND FEATURES OF THE WORKFORCE

Because a group as difficult to identify as clinical researchers cannot be accurately measured, we have attempted only the most general estimates of the size and characteristics of the workforce. According to data collected by the American Medical Association, research was the primary professional activity of 14,434 M.D.s and M.D.-Ph.D.s in 1997.[6] If the percentage of clinical researchers in this pool were the same as for the M.D.s and M.D.-Ph.D.s supported by the NIH and AHRQ in 1997 (34 percent for the two agencies combined), the number of physicians in the clinical research workforce would have been 4,908. Add 14,618 Ph.D.s from the fields traditionally associated with clinical research working in science in 1997 (see Table G-6), and the estimated total size of the workforce that year was 19,526. Of course, this figure may well be an underestimate; it does not include dentists or other health care doctorates active in clinical research, about whom little is known, or Ph.D.s trained in the basic biomedical or behavioral and social sciences, some of whom are part of the clinical research workforce, at least part of the time.

The two major groups of investigators in the clinical research workforce are quite different in character, except for their age.[7-12] In 1997 the median age of physicians whose primary activity was research was approximately 47.8, just under that of Ph.D.s conducting clinical research, whose median age was 48. Women were more likely to be found among the Ph.D.s conducting clinical research (52.7 percent) than among physician-scientists (17.6 percent). The same is true of underrepresented minorities. In 1997, 7.8 percent of Ph.D.s conducting clinical research were underrepresented minorities, more than double the estimate for U.S.-trained physician-scientists (3.5 percent).

Physician-scientists also differ from physicians in practice and other nonresearch activities. In 1997 they were two years older than the rest of the physician workforce, whose median age was 45.8. The portion of the physician workforce outside of research also included slightly more women (22.1 percent) and nearly twice as many underrepresented minorities (7.1 percent).

The relative roles of M.D.s and Ph.D.s in the clinical research workforce appear to have changed considerably from what they were a few decades ago. If the proportion of physicians conducting clinical research had been the same in the mid-1970s as today, there would have been more physicians than Ph.D.s in the clinical research workforce of 1975. By 1997 it was likely that the opposite was the case (see Figure 4-1).

---

[6] Pasko, Thomas, and Bradley Seidman. *Physician Characteristics and Distribution in the US, 1999.* Chicago: American Medical Association, 1999.

[7] Ibid.

[8] Unpublished tabulation from the Survey of Doctorate Recipients; on file in the archives of the Academies.

[9] Table G-6.

[10] Pasko, Thomas, and Bradley Seidman. *Physician Characteristics and Distribution in the US, 1999.* Chicago: American Medical Association, 1999.

[11] Unpublished tabulation from the Association of American Medical Colleges, Minority Physician Database; on file in the archives of the Academies.

[12] Pasko, Thomas, and Bradley Seidman. *Physician Characteristics and Distribution in the US, 1999.* Chicago: American Medical Association, 1999.

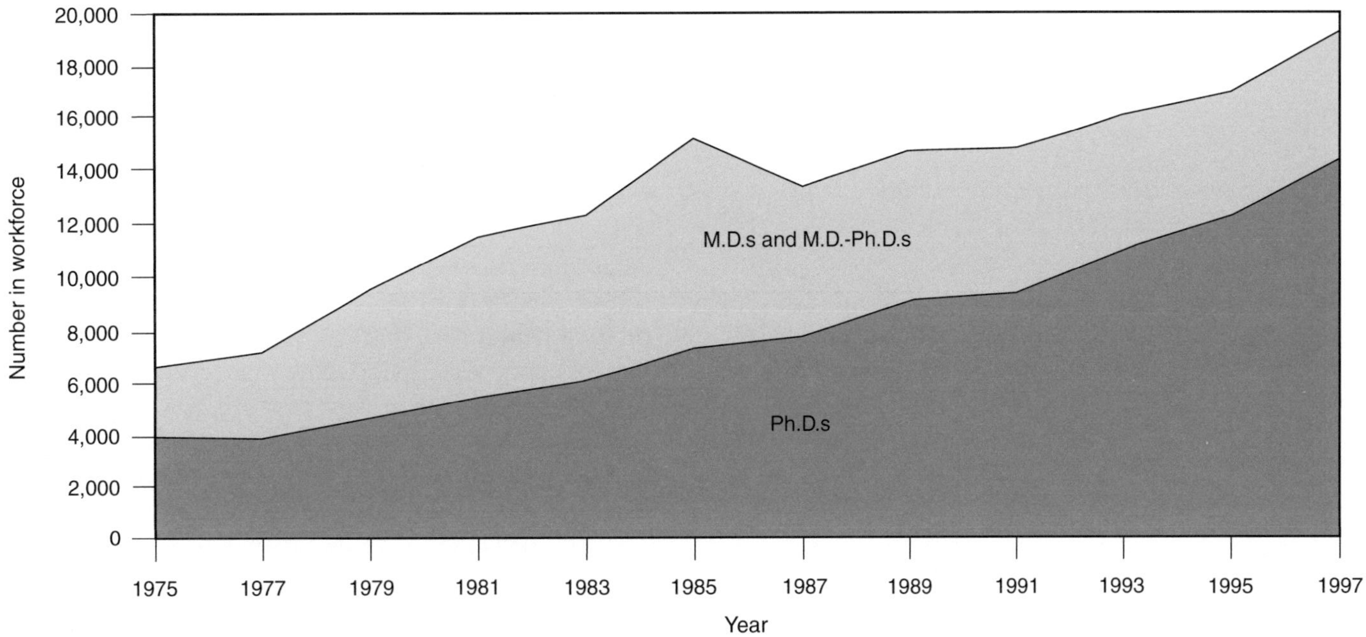

FIGURE 4-1 Trends in the composition of the clinical research workforce. The number of M.D-Ph.D.s is estimated, using the assumption that 34 percent of physicians whose primary professional activity is research are conducting clinical research. SOURCES: Data are from the Survey of Doctorate Recipients and the American Medical Association, *Physician Characteristics and Distribution in the United States,* various years.

From 1975 to 1997, the number of Ph.D.s from fields traditionally associated with clinical research who were working in science more than quadrupled, increasing from 3,515 to 14,618.

THE ECONOMICS OF CLINICAL RESEARCH

When concerns about the declining role of M.D.s in the research workforce began to emerge 20 years ago,[13] many attributed the trend to the difference between the salaries of academic and private-practice physicians. Since then the disincentives for physicians and other health care doctorates to pursue research careers have grown. These include increasing levels of educational indebtedness, continuing discrepancies between research training stipends and salaries paid to medical residents, limited time for research, and salaries of investigators.

Except for graduates of dual-degree (e.g., M.D.-Ph.D. or D.D.S.-Ph.D.) programs, most physicians and dentists today begin their professional careers with sizable educational debts. From 1990 to 1997, the average medical school debt of M.D. graduates increased more than 50 percent, from almost $41,000 (in 1997 dollars) to just over $64,000.[14] For underrepresented minorities, the debt burden is generally even more. The average medical school debt reported by minority students graduating in 1997 was nearly $68,500, roughly $5,000 more than for white and Asian students.[15]

The amount of medical school debt for M.D.-Ph.D. students graduating in 1997 was considerably less and lower still for participants in the NRSA Medical Scientist Training Program; the latter had a mean debt of about $13,600 (Table 4-3).

Levels of educational debt for dental students are higher than those in medicine, but this debt increased

[13] Wyngaarden, James B. "The Clinical Investigator as an Endangered Species." *New England Journal of Medicine* 301, December 1979, 1254–59.

[14] Unpublished tabulation from the Association of American Medical Colleges, Student and Applicant Information Management System and the National Research Council; on file in the archives of the Academies.

[15] Unpublished tabulation from the Association of American Medical Colleges, Student and Applicant Information Management System; available from the archives of the Academies.

TABLE 4-3 Medical School Debt Reported by 1997 Graduates

	MD-Ph.D.s			
	MSTP[a]	Non-MSTP	Subtotal	All others
All graduates	178	324	502	15,426
Mean	$13,598	$44,787	$33,728	$64,052
Graduates with debt	71	205	276	10,723
Mean	$26,239	$60,299	$51,537	$77,582

[a] Participants in the NRSA Medical Scientist Training Program.

SOURCE: Data are from the Association of American Medical Colleges, Student and Applicant Information Management System.

at a slower rate in the 1990s. In 1997, graduating dentists reported nearly $75,000 in dental school debt, up from just over $62,000 (in 1997 dollars) in 1990.[16,17]

Although health care professionals are permitted to postpone payments on their student loans during NRSA or other authorized research training programs, this option may not be as widely used as intended. In informal polls of research fellows at major Boston and San Francisco teaching hospitals, our committee found that a large majority of fellows took advantage of loan deferments, but a number of others were not aware they qualified for a deferment.[18,19] Even with deferment of their loan payments, research training generally entails financial sacrifice for young physicians. Despite the significant increase in NRSA stipends in 1999, payments for physicians in research training are generally less than the salaries paid to medical residents. Following the third year of residency, for example, when many young physicians have their first opportunity for postdoctoral research training, the NRSA stipend is $36,036, nearly $3,000 less than the average payment for medical residents with the same experience.[20,21]

After their research training, physicians face still further obstacles in establishing research careers. First, they have to find—or negotiate—time for research, an increasingly difficult matter, particularly for those working in highly competitive health care markets. According to a 1997 study of the activities of medical school faculty, new faculty members in the most competitive health care markets were more likely to have patient care duties, spend more time teaching, and publish fewer papers than their peers in other parts of the country. Even in their own institutions, junior faculty in the most competitive health care markets had greater teaching responsibilities and were more likely to be assigned to patient care duties than their more senior colleagues. In light of these findings, the study's authors cautioned that protected time for new clinical faculty to conduct research is threatened by the growing competition in health care.[22]

Another obstacle for physician-investigators has been the limitation on salaries for NIH-funded investigators that Congress imposed in 1990.[23] (Although not required to do so, AHRQ has followed the NIH policy and has restricted the salaries of its investigators as well.)[24] Now set at $141,300, the maximum allowable salary for researchers supported by either agency is less than most medical school faculty members earn. During the 1997-1998 academic year, physicians serving as assistant professors in medical school clinical departments received an average base salary of $127,800 and associate and full professors received $151,600 and $181,000, respectively.[25] While most investigators

[16] American Association of Dental Schools, Survey of Dental School Seniors—1998 Graduating Class. Washington, D.C.: AADS, 1998.

[17] Unpublished tabulation from the National Research Council; available from the archives of the Academies.

[18] Goldman, Lee. Department of Medicine, University of California, San Francisco School of Medicine. Personal communication, January 1999.

[19] Hiatt, Howard. Department of Medicine, Harvard Medical School. Personal communication, March 1999.

[20] "National Research Service Award (NRSA) Stipend Increase." *NIH Guide for Grants and Contracts*, 19 November 1998. Available: http://grants.nih.gov/grants/guide/index.html.

[21] Association of American Medical Colleges. *AAMC Data Book: Statistical Information Related to Medical Schools and Teaching Hospitals*. Washington, D.C.: AAMC, 1999.

[22] Campbell, Eric G., Joel S. Weissman, and David Blumenthal. "Relationship Between Market Competition and the Activities and Attitudes of Medical School Faculty." *JAMA* 278, no. 3 (1997): 222-26.

[23] "Salary Limitation on Grants, Cooperative Agreements and Contracts." *NIH Guide for Grants and Contracts*, 6 January 2000. Available: http://grants.nih.gov/grants/guide/index.html.

[24] Drott, Greta. Agency for Healthcare Quality and Research. Personal communication, July 1999.

[25] Association of American Medical Colleges. *AAMC Data Book: Statistical Information Related to Medical Schools and Teaching Hospitals*. Washington, D.C.: AAMC, 1999.

spend less than full-time in research, their base compensation must still be calibrated to the salary cap. So, for example, a faculty member conducting research half-time cannot draw more than $70,650 in salary from an NIH or AHRQ grant. As a result, medical schools and their faculty must often seek supplementary funds from other sources to carry out federally sponsored clinical research.

THE CHANGING ROLE OF THE NATIONAL RESEARCH SERVICE AWARD PROGRAM

Other than M.D.-Ph.D.s, whose numbers have been steadily growing, as shown in Figure 4-2, the number of medical students receiving research training has remained relatively constant during the 1990s. Over the same time period, M.D.s participating in postdoctoral NRSA programs declined by more than 20 percent, from 2,228 to 1,775 (Figure 4-3).

In contrast to their declining participation in NRSA training programs overall, increasing numbers of M.D.s and other health care doctorates have obtained research training and experience through mentored career development awards (Figure 4-4). From 1988 to 1997, career development awards granted to physicians and dentists increased by 62 percent, from 674 to 1,092. It is not clear what accounts for the upsurge in career development awards to health care doctorates, but the compensation that accompanies these awards is likely a factor. In contrast to postdoctoral NRSA awards, which require the recipient to be in full-time training and provide a maximum stipend of $41,268,[26] salaries for mentored career development awards generally range from $50,000 to $75,000 for a commitment of 75 percent time (although a few NIH institutes provide up to the maximum allowable under the salary cap, $141,300).[27] In addition, career development awards

[26] "National Research Service Award (NRSA) Stipend Increase," *NIH Guide for Grants and Contracts*, 19 November 1998. Available: http://grants.nih.gov/grants/guide/index.html.

[27] National Institutes of Health. Office of Extramural Research. "Extramural Training Career Development Awards," and from relevant NIH institute links. Online. Available: http://grants.nih.gov/training/careerdevelopment awards.htm. Accessed 8 December 1999.

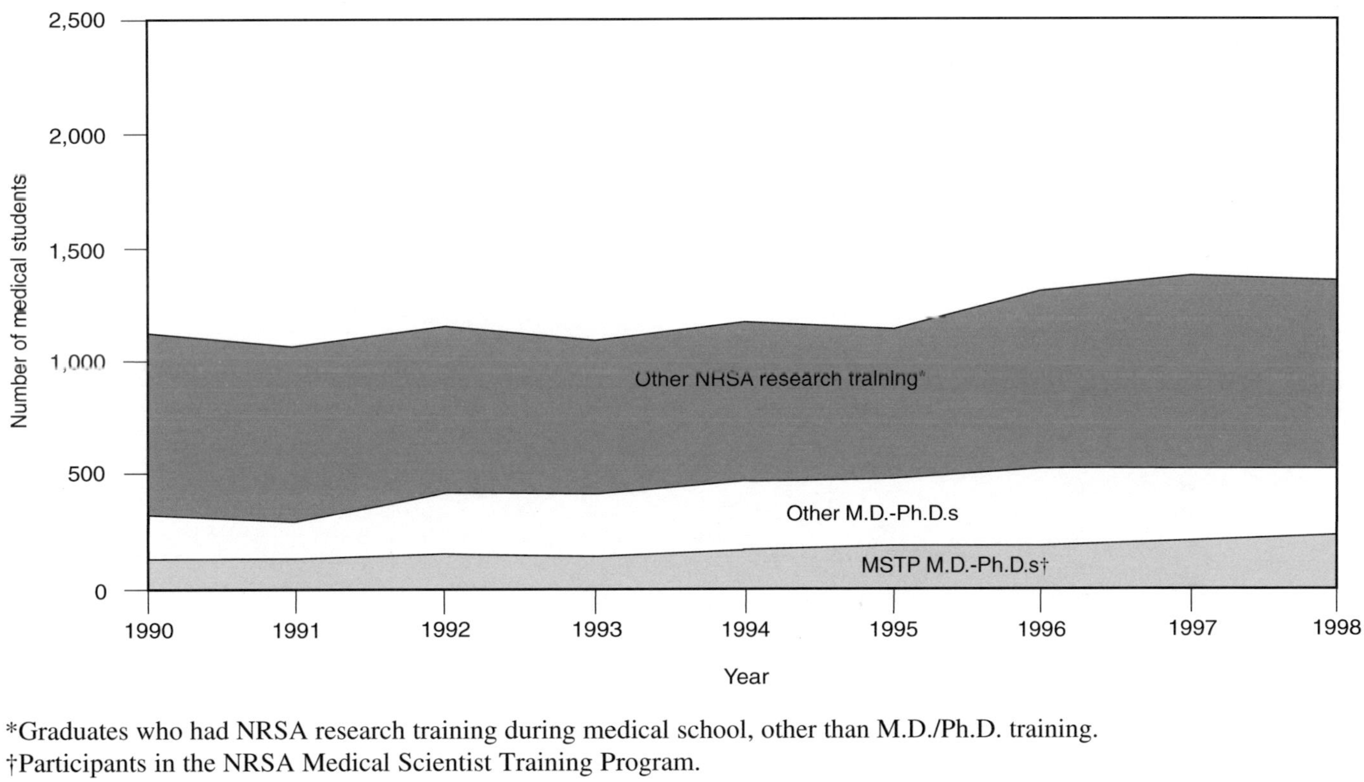

*Graduates who had NRSA research training during medical school, other than M.D./Ph.D. training.
†Participants in the NRSA Medical Scientist Training Program.

FIGURE 4-2 Students receiving various types of research training during medical school. Some M.D.-Ph.D.s participated in the NRSA Medical Scientist Training Program (MSTP); other NRSA participants generally received short-term research training. SOURCES: Data are from the Association of American Medical Colleges, Student and Applicant Information Management System, and the NIH Trainee and Fellow File.

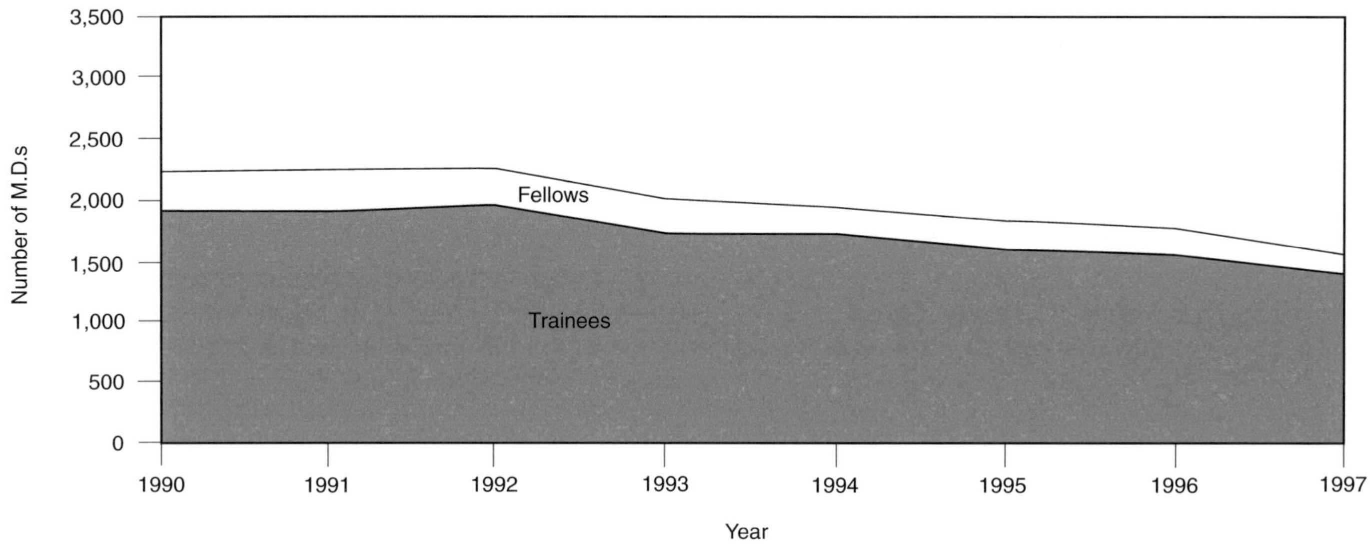

FIGURE 4-3 Physicians in postdoctoral NRSA training. SOURCE: Data are from the NIH Trainee and Fellow File.

include funds for research expenses, usually between $10,000 and $25,000.

In recent years the NIH has increasingly encouraged the use of career development awards for clinical research training. When the agency unveiled three new grant programs to foster the training and retention of clinical investigators in 1998, all three programs took the form of career development awards.[28] In the fall of

[28] National Institutes of Health. "New Initiative in Clinical Research Training and Career Development." *NIH Backgrounder.* Bethesda, Md.: NIH, 6 March 1998.

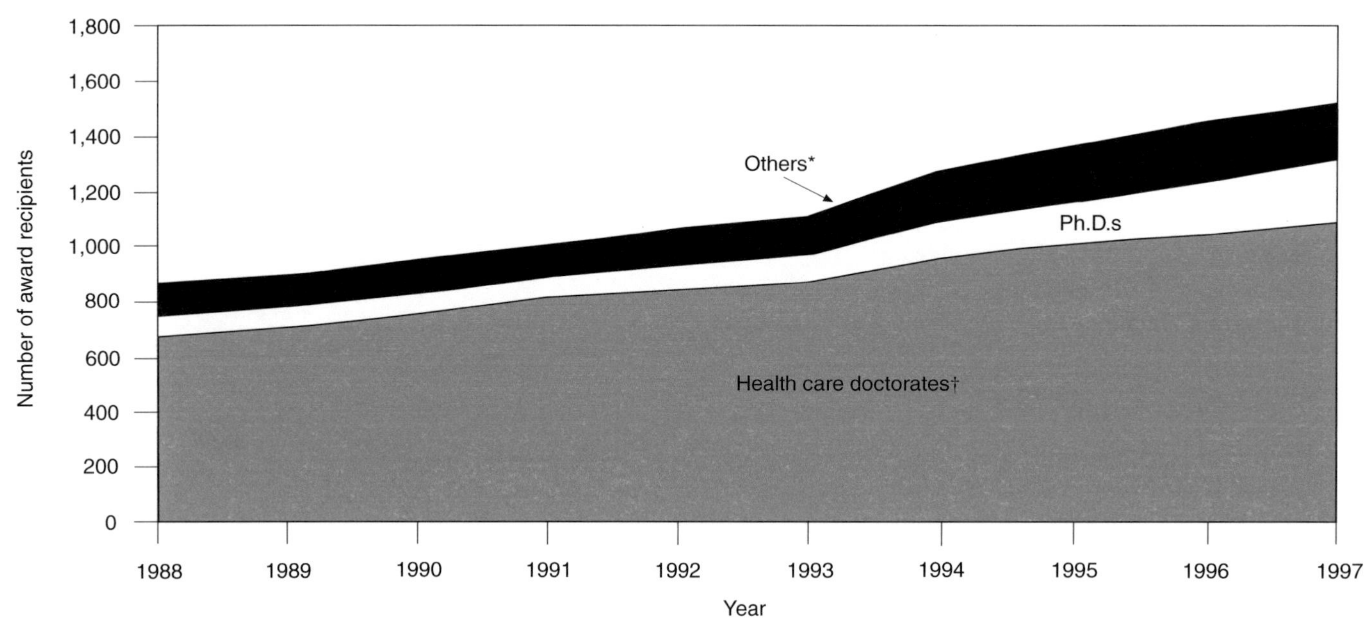

*Includes dual-degree holders (M.D./Ph.D.s, D.D.S./Ph.D.s), veterinarians, and others.
†Includes physicians and dentists.

FIGURE 4-4 Recipients of mentored career development awards by degree type. Mentored career development award mechanisms include the K01, K08, K11, K14, K15, K17, K20 and K21. SOURCE: Data are from the NIH IMPAC System.

1999 the AHRQ followed suit and offered career development awards for clinicians committed to careers in health services research.[29]

Given their financial advantages, dual-degree programs would seem to be another attractive option for health care professionals seeking clinical research training. To date, the NIH has developed several types of dual-degree training: (1) the Medical Scientist Training Program, (2) individual M.D.-Ph.D. fellowships, and (3) the Dental Scientist Training Program. The oldest and largest of these is the Medical Scientist Training Program (MSTP), established by the National Institute of General Medical Sciences in 1964. Today, the education and research training of nearly 900 medical students are supported by MSTP training grants to 38 medical schools and universities.[30,31] Fellowships for M.D.-Ph.D. training are a more recent development, instituted in 1989 by the National Institute of Mental Health, the National Institute on Alcohol Abuse and Alcoholism, and the National Institute on Drug Abuse to encourage dual-degree training in the areas of mental health, behavior, and neuroscience. The fellowship program is much smaller in scale, supporting about 40 students a year.[32] The latest type of dual-degree training to be introduced is the Dental Scientist Training Program (DSTP), which was created following the recommendations from the committee preceding ours. Since the first DSTP training grants were awarded in 1996, the program has grown to support roughly 10 students in three dental schools, and the National Institute of Dental and Craniofacial Research has also introduced an individual fellowship award for dental students in dual-degree training.[33,34]

Each of these avenues for NRSA dual-degree training provides participating students with tuition support and stipends while they pursue professional and doctoral training, allowing them to earn two degrees in roughly seven years and graduate with very little—or no—educational debt. Indeed, the difference in the indebtedness between recent M.D.s and their classmates who received NIH support through the Medical Scientist Training Program is striking. Of the 178 MSTP students who graduated in 1997, just over 60 percent (107) reported no medical school debt (Table 4-3); of those with educational debt, the average amount owed was just over $26,200, about one-third of that reported by their medical school classmates graduating with the M.D. alone (who reported owing more than $77,500).

Yet despite the attractions of M.D.-Ph.D. programs, relatively few participants receive research training in clinical research methods; neither do they go on to conduct clinical research. A 1996 analysis of the fields of study chosen by MSTP participants found that nearly 60 percent of graduates from the late 1980s and early 1990s received their Ph.D.s in five basic science fields: biochemistry, neuroscience, molecular biology, cell biology, and pharmacology.[35] Further, in their subsequent research careers, MSTP graduates focused almost entirely on laboratory-oriented research and sought NIH funding for such research projects at the same rate as Ph.D.s.

This emphasis on laboratory-oriented research stems, in part, from the conventional organization of M.D.-Ph.D. training. Traditionally, dual-degree programs have encouraged and in many cases directed their students toward doctoral study in the basic biomedical sciences. More recently, however, the National Institute of General Medical Sciences has recommended that institutions provide broad opportunities for M.D.-Ph.D. training, recognizing that restrictions on student choice of training areas may limit their subsequent fields of investigation.

In early 1997 the National Institute of General Medical Sciences issued new guidelines for its Medical Scientist Training Program, urging the medical schools with such training grants to extend their programs to give students "a breadth of doctoral research training opportunities," in fields including computer science,

[29] "Mentored Clinical Scientist Development Award," *NIH Guide for Grants and Contracts*, 11 November 1999. Available: http://grants.nih.gov/grants/guide/index.html.

[30] National Institutes of Health. National Institute of General Medical Sciences. *The Careers and Professional Activities of Graduates of the NIGMS Medical Scientist Training Program.* Bethesda, Md.: NIH, September 1998.

[31] National Institutes of Health. National Institute of General Medical Sciences. "Medical Scientist Training Program (MSTP) Institutions." Online. Available: http://www.nih.gov/nigms/funding/mstp.html. Accessed 3 March 2000.

[32] Unpublished tabulation from the NIH IMPAC System; available from the archives of the Academies.

[33] Lipton, James. National Institute of Dental and Craniofacial Research. Personal communication, July 1999.

[34] "Individual Predoctoral Dental Scientist Fellowship," *NIH Guide for Grants and Contracts,* 15 August 1997. Available: http://grants.nih.gov/grants/guide/index/html.

[35] Sutton, Jennifer, and Charles D. Killian. "The M.D.-Ph.D. Researcher—What Species of Investigator?" *Academic Medicine* 71 (May 1996): 454–59.

the social and behavioral sciences, economics, epidemiology, public health, bioengineering, biostatistics, and bioethics.[36] So far, most M.D.-Ph.D. programs have been slow to respond. An examination of catalogs, brochures, and other program materials at the start of the 1999-2000 academic year revealed that few programs had expanded their offerings. Almost 60 percent still advise prospective dual-degree students that their options for pursuing a Ph.D. are limited to the biological, chemical, and physical sciences; other programs generally offer only one or two choices outside these fields.

To adapt to the new National Institute of General Medical Sciences policy, some M.D.-Ph.D. programs may need to expand their rosters to encompass additional fields of study in the medical school, such as the Ph.D. programs in clinical research that Johns Hopkins and UCLA have introduced.[37] Others may opt to forge ties with doctoral programs in departments outside of the medical school, as the University of North Carolina has done with the Department of Epidemiology in its School of Public Health.[38] Still others may seek to establish links to neighboring universities, as Emory has with Georgia Tech for training in bioengineering.[39]

Finally, the extent to which Medical Scientist Training Programs sponsored by the National Institute of General Medical Sciences offer their students the opportunity to earn Ph.D.s in a broad range of fields in addition to the basic biomedical sciences may influence other dual-degree programs. For example, because the M.D.-Ph.D. fellowships sponsored by the National Institute of Mental Health, National Institute on Drug Abuse, and National Institute on Alcohol Abuse and Alcoholism are generally available only to those enrolled in existing M.D.-Ph.D. programs, there is little opportunity for these fellows to obtain many of the research skills that facilitate clinical research related to behavior and mental health. Almost all recipients of these fellowships so far have graduated with Ph.D.s in basic biomedical disciplines, rather than in the behavioral or social sciences.[40]

As in the basic biomedical and behavioral and social sciences, Ph.D. production in the fields associated with clinical research has expanded. Indeed, the number of clinical science Ph.D.s has grown at a rate much faster than in the biomedical or behavioral sciences. In 1997, 1,349 Ph.D.s were awarded in clinical research-related fields, almost six times the number in 1975 (see Table G-3).

Meanwhile, the numbers of women, minorities, and noncitizens earning degrees have all increased. In a pattern of growth nearly identical to the behavioral and social sciences, the percentage of women earning doctoral degrees in clinical fields has more than doubled since 1975, growing from 31.3 percent in 1975 to 64.5 percent in 1997. The share of Ph.D.s earned by minorities, furthermore, increased at a more rapid pace than in any other field in this study, from 0.9 percent in 1975 to 5.9 percent in 1997. Today, the clinical sciences rank above the biomedical but below the behavioral sciences in the percentage of doctoral degrees earned by minorities.

The percentage of clinical science Ph.D.s awarded to noncitizens has always been relatively high; in 1975, for example, temporary-visa holders earned a greater share of doctoral degrees awarded in the clinical sciences (9.1 percent) than in the biomedical sciences (8.3 percent). Since then the fraction of clinical science Ph.D.s awarded to temporary-visa holders has doubled, growing to 18.3 percent in 1997, just below that in biomedical fields.

Time to degree has also increased in the clinical sciences, and those earning Ph.D.s are older than ever before. Today, clinical science Ph.D.s typically earn their degrees 10 years after beginning graduate study (median time to degree, as measured from entry into post-baccalaureate study) at a median age of 38.4. In 1975 the median time to degree was seven years, and the median age of Ph.D.s was less than 32.

Ph.D.s in nursing present a special situation; on average, they complete their degrees much later in life. In many cases, this may result from pursuing a Ph.D. part-time. Even those receiving NRSA funds, which require

[36] Described in memorandum to NIGMS Training Grant Program Directors from John Norvell, April 29, 1997.

[37] Association of American Medical Colleges. *For the Health of the Public: Ensuring the Future of Clinical Research.* Washington, D.C.: AAMC, 2000.

[38] University of North Carolina at Chapel Hill School of Medicine. M.D.-Ph.D. Program. "Research." Online. Available: http://www.med.unc.edu/mdphd/researchINFO.htm. Accessed 5 March 2000.

[39] Emory School of Medicine. M.D.-Ph.D. Program. "Program Information." Online. Available: http://omesa.medadm.emory.edu/MDPHD/program.html. Accessed 1 February 2000.

[40] Unpublished tabulation from the NIH Trainee and Fellow File and the Survey of Earned Doctorates; available from the archives of the Academies.

full-time study, however, are generally past 40 by the time they finish their studies. The median age at which an NRSA recipient completes a nursing Ph.D. is over 41 years, in marked contrast to the basic biomedical sciences, where NRSA recipients complete their Ph.D.s at a median age of 30, and the behavioral and social sciences receive their degrees at age 32.[41]

The advanced age of nursing Ph.D.s stems, in part, from the norms of the profession, which encourages its members to acquire considerable professional experience before seeking research training. Although this practice ensures professional expertise, later research training inevitably limits the length of an individual's research career. The advanced age of nursing Ph.D.s also poses a staffing challenge for nursing school administrators. The median age of nursing school faculty is now 50, and many nursing school deans report concerns about their abilities to replace retiring faculty.[42]

IMPLICATIONS AND RECOMMENDATIONS

Overall, the clinical research workforce lags well behind both the basic biomedical and the behavioral and social science workforces in size. Given the apparently ample supply of both biomedical and behavioral researchers, however, the significance of this difference in workforce dimensions is not entirely clear.

Within the clinical research workforce itself, the considerable growth in the number of research doctorates awarded in fields related to clinical research since 1975 has yielded an abundant supply of Ph.D.s. Other than the advanced age of Ph.D.s in nursing, the committee finds little cause for concern in the training and supply of clinical research Ph.D.s.

Over the same time period, however, the number of physician-investigators has declined, as fewer physicians have pursued research training and established research careers. The evidence suggests that the decline in health care doctorates in the clinical research workforce is due in large measure to the economic disincentives associated with NRSA research training and the conduct of federally funded research.

Because those who interact with patients often bring great understanding and awareness of the health needs of the public to clinical research, the diminishing role played by physicians affects the capacity of the clinical research workforce to sustain a program of research that addresses the nation's needs. If this pool of investigators dwindles further, it is possible that the NIH—which has depended on physician-investigators to initiate much of the clinical research it supports—may not be able to maintain its clinical research portfolio at current levels.

The NIH, the Agency for Healthcare Research and Quality, and the Health Resources and Services Administration should pay increased attention to the training of underrepresented minorities for the clinical research workforce. The number of minority students earning Ph.D.s in clinical science fields has increased since 1975, but this trend must accelerate if the workforce is to better reflect the nation's increasing diversity and to meet the nation's changing health needs. The number of minority physicians and dentists in research cannot be easily determined, but the estimates for physicians, at least, suggest that underrepresented minorities pursue research careers at about half the rate they choose other careers in medicine.

Future analyses of this workforce would be improved by more data on the training and careers of physicians and other health care doctorates who conduct clinical research, as well as by a better understanding of the role played by Ph.D.s from fields other than those traditionally associated with clinical research.

Recommendation 4-1. The NIH, the Agency for Healthcare Research and Quality, and the Health Resources and Services Administration should intensify their efforts to train and retain physicians in clinical research until the decline in the numbers has been reversed and the clinical research workforce includes substantially more M.D.s and other health care doctorates than is now the case.

Without adequate numbers of physicians and other health care doctorates, the research conducted by the clinical research workforce will almost surely fail to fully reflect the nation's needs. The committee commends the NIH's introduction of a new series of career development awards to enhance the clinical research training of physicians and other health care professionals and recommends that the agency carefully monitor and report on the outcomes of these new initiatives. In addition, the committee urges the

[41] Unpublished tabulation from the NIH Trainee and Fellow File and the Survey of Earned Doctorates; available from the archives of the Academies.

[42] American Association of Colleges of Nursing. *1998-1999 Salaries of Instructional and Administrative Nursing Faculty in Baccalaureate and Graduate Programs in Nursing*. Washington, D.C.: AACN, 1999.

NIH, the Agency for Healthcare Research and Quality, and the Health Resources and Services Administration to consider additional measures to bolster the training and retention of health care doctorates in clinical research, including those described in the following recommendations.

Recommendation 4-2. The NIH, the Agency for Healthcare Research and Quality, and the Health Resources and Services Administration should substantially increase opportunities for dual-degree training in fields related to clinical research.

The committee urges the agencies to work together to substantially increase opportunities for dual-degree training (whether M.D.-Ph.D., M.D.-M.P.H., or dual-degree programs targeted to dentists and other health care doctorates) in fields related to clinical research, such as epidemiology, psychology, and health services research.

Recommendation 4-3. The NIH, the Agency for Healthcare Research and Quality, and the Health Resources and Services Administration should take steps to reduce the economic barriers to clinical research careers faced by physicians, dentists, and other health care doctorates.

The committee urges the agencies to work together to (1) ensure that physicians and dentists in postdoctoral research training are fully informed of their options for loan deferment and (2) seek legislative authority to establish extramural loan repayment programs for those who pursue clinical research training and careers. In addition, the committee urges the NIH and the Agency for Healthcare Quality and Research to consider seeking legislative authority to raise the salary cap above current levels for physicians and other health care doctorates conducting clinical research.

Recommendation 4-4. The NIH, the Agency for Healthcare Research and Quality, and the Health Resources and Services Administration should take additional steps to improve their understanding of the training and career paths of clinical investigators.

Since the NIH began to monitor the number of clinical research grants it awards, its efforts have yielded some important new data on the clinical research workforce. Still, information on the training and career paths of physicians, dentists, and other health care doctorates is too limited to permit detailed analyses of the clinical research workforce.

Recommendation 4-5. There should be no growth in the aggregate number of Ph.D.s awarded annually in the fields traditionally associated with clinical research.

Given the considerable growth in the number of research doctorates awarded in clinical science fields since 1975, and the resulting expansion of the Ph.D. portion of the clinical research workforce, the committee finds no reason for Ph.D. production to increase outside of dual-degree programs.

Recommendation 4-6. The National Institute of Nursing Research should emphasize research training programs that foster earlier entry into research careers.

Delayed research training inevitably limits the length of an investigator's research career and affects the supply of nursing faculty. The National Institute of Nursing Research may wish to consider redirecting a portion of its NRSA funds to programs targeting students entering the nursing profession (such as B.A.-to-Ph.D. programs) and recent nursing graduates.

Recommendation 4-7. The NIH, the Agency for Healthcare Research and Quality, and the Health Resources and Services Administration should increase their efforts to identify and support programs that encourage and prepare underrepresented minority students for careers in clinical research.

Although the number of underrepresented minority men and women earning Ph.D.s in the clinical sciences has grown over the last few decades, the NIH and its fellow agencies should increase their efforts to ensure that these trends accelerate. In addition, the NIH, the Agency for Healthcare Research and Quality, and the Health Resources and Services Administration should intensify their efforts to increase the percentage of minority physicians in research, which appears to be about half that of other careers in medicine.

5

Crosscutting Issues in Research Training

In addition to reviewing the size of the research workforce in the biomedical, behavioral, and clinical sciences, and assessing the likely needs for future investigators, the committee appraised the effectiveness of the research training activities sponsored by the National Institutes of Health, the Agency for Healthcare Research and Quality, and the Health Resources and Services Administration. Although the preceding chapters examine many of these issues, the committee found that a number of the questions were recurring ones, arising in nearly every field of research training:

- What are the best ways to develop a research workforce that is representative of the nation and fully addresses the population's health needs?
- Would research training be more effective if the NRSA program were better coordinated with other federal funding mechanisms for students and young investigators?
- How should stipend levels and other forms of compensation for those in training be set?
- What role should the National Institutes of Health (NIH) and other federal agencies play in providing research training to students from outside the U.S.?

DEVELOPING A RESEARCH WORKFORCE THAT REFLECTS THE NATION AND ADDRESSES ITS HEALTH NEEDS

Despite enormous advances in the health of Americans during the 20th century, the health status of the nation's minorities at every stage of life is much worse than that of the rest of the population. Research into the reasons for these disparities has generally targeted factors such as income, education, and occupation and has shown that these factors have a great influence on health. Still, race has been found to have an effect on health independent of socioeconomic status, and those who have studied health disparities find that cultural influences, social factors, and racism all play a role.[1] As the population of the nation grows more diverse, it is crucial that the research workforce increase its focus on those disparities.

Over the past 20 years, the federal government has devoted substantial effort and funds to increasing the representation of minorities in the research workforce. During that time, both the number and the percentage of science Ph.D.s earned by underrepresented minorities have grown (see Tables G-1, G-2, and G-3). The rate of growth has been slow, however, and the percentage of minorities in research remains less than in the health professions and substantially less than in society at large (see Table 5-1).

The situation is much the same for the NIH and its fellow agencies in the Department of Health and Human Services. None of the many initiatives undertaken by these agencies to date—either within or outside the NRSA program—appear to have had a major impact on the diversity of the health research workforce.

A 1993 report on NIH's programs found "a modest effect" on the number of underrepresented minorities among the agency's grant recipients.[2] That analysis,

[1] Williams, David R., Risa Lavizzo-Mourey, and Rueben C. Warren. "The Concept of Race and Health Status in America." *Public Health Reports* 109 (1994): 26-41.

[2] National Institutes of Health. Office of Research on Minority Health. *Assessment of NIH Minority Research/Training Programs: Phase 1*. Bethesda, Md.: NIH, 1993.

TABLE 5-1 Racial and Ethnic Distribution of Selected Populations, 1997 (percent)

	African American	Hispanic	Native American	Asian	White
U.S. population[a]	12.1	10.9	0.7	3.6	72.7
Ph.D. recipients in the basic biomedical sciences[b]	2.7	3.4	0.2	18.2	72.9
Ph.D. recipients in the behavioral and social sciences[b]	5.0	4.7	0.7	4.7	78.7
Ph.D. recipients in the clinical sciences	5.1	3.0	0.6	9.7	80.3
NRSA trainees and fellows[b]	6.2	5.1	0.6	17.1	70.9
M.D.-Ph.D. graduates	3.6	4.0	0.6	18.5	72.8
Medical school graduates	7.3	5.9	0.6	15.9	68.1
Dental school graduates	5.4	5.5	0.2	18.2	70.2

[a] The resident population of the mainland United States, estimated from the 1990 census.
[b] U.S. citizens and permanent residents.

SOURCES: Data on Ph.D.s, NRSA trainees and fellows, and M.D.-Ph.D.s are from the Survey of Earned Doctorates, the NIH IMPAC System, and the Association of American Medical Colleges, respectively. Data on the U.S. population are from the U.S. Census Bureau, Population Estimates Program. Data on medical school graduates are from the Association of American Medical Colleges, *AAMC Data Book*, 1999. Data on dental school graduates are from the American Dental Association, Survey Center, *1997-1998 Survey of Predoctoral Dental Educational Institutions.*

however, studied the combined effects of all NIH programs and was hampered by limited data, which led to recommendations for improved data collection and separate evaluations of each of the agency's major programs. Since then the NIH has completed a follow-up study of undergraduates who participated in the Minority Access to Research Careers (MARC) program, an NRSA initiative and the NIH's largest program devoted to building the diversity of the research workforce.[3]

Still, like the agency-wide assessment before it, the MARC program evaluation found little change in the number of science Ph.D.s earned by graduates of colleges that received MARC training grants. Nearly half the MARC participants since the program began in 1977 went on to advanced study, but twice as many earned medical or dental degrees as Ph.D.s.

Other NIH programs aimed at increasing the diversity of the research workforce include bridge grants, which link major research universities to colleges with significant minority enrollments[4] and research supplements for investigators who recruit minority students and fellows to work as research assistants on their projects.[5] Both initiatives are less than a decade old, however, and their effectiveness has yet to be assessed.

Without information on the relative success of federal programs for increasing the diversity of the research workforce, it is impossible to advocate one approach over another or to determine which program characteristics are the most significant. Nonetheless, several points merit further attention. First, since MARC participants have shown a greater inclination to earn a medical or dental degree than a Ph.D.,[6] the program's effectiveness might be heightened by further increasing its emphasis on research careers. In addition, because some colleges and universities (the University of Maryland, Baltimore County, for example)[7] are particularly successful at encouraging minority students to pursue research careers, it would be

[3] National Institutes of Health. National Institute of General Medical Sciences. *A Study of the Minority Access to Research Careers Honors Undergraduate Research Training Program.* Bethesda, Md.: NIH, 1995.

[4] "Initiatives for Minority Students: Bridges to the Future," *NIH Guide for Grants and Contracts*, 24 January 1992. Available: http://grants.nih.gov/grants/guide/index/html.

[5] "Research Supplements for Underrepresented Minorities," *NIH Guide for Grants and Contracts*, 24 January 1992. Available: http://grants.nih.gov/grants/guide/index.html.

[6] National Institutes of Health. National Institute of General Medical Sciences. *A Study of the Minority Access to Research Careers Honors Undergraduate Research Training Program.* Bethesda, Md.: NIH, 1995.

[7] Maton, Kenneth I., Freeman A. Hrabowski III, and Carol L. Schmitt. "African-American College Students Excelling in the Sciences: College and Post-College Outcomes in the Meyerhoff Scholars Program." *Journal of Research in Science Teaching*, in press.

useful for the NIH to identify the factors common to the most effective MARC programs and ensure that they are replicated wherever possible.

A 1998 revision of the MARC program announcement directed institutions that receive these training grants to establish measurable goals and specific objectives for their programs, monitor their progress, and be prepared to demonstrate the benefits of MARC funding on measures such as student recruitment, retention, and career outcomes.[8] Whether this policy change will make a difference in the composition of the research workforce is unlikely to be evident for a number of years.

Ultimately, unless larger numbers of minority students enter college prepared to pursue classes in science and math, it is not likely that the MARC program (or any other programs aimed at college or graduate students) will ever have more than a limited effect on the diversity of the research workforce. Though the NIH has not traditionally played a major role in secondary education, its responsibility for ensuring diversity in the research workforce requires that it consider doing so.

Success in college and graduate school science and math generally requires a rigorous high school background.[9] Science magnet schools often excel in this area, and other approaches have been successful as well. For example, in the New York City public schools involved in the "Gateway to Higher Education" program, participating students take all their classes together, participate in study groups, and have an extended and enriched school day and an 11-month school year. Since the program's inception in 1986, its graduates have completed high school with an average of three advanced placement courses, and 97 percent have gone on to 4-year colleges. By the fourth year of college, 59 percent reported plans for a science-based career, such as medicine, computer science, engineering, or research.[10]

Investigators from minority backgrounds will not, of course, necessarily pursue research on health disparities. Nor should it be assumed that only investigators from minority backgrounds can effectively conduct such research. Yet those from minority groups are more likely than others to be aware of the health problems of disadvantaged populations and, if they choose to address such problems in their research, the committee believes that they are likely to do so with great insight, motivation, and persistence.

Many research training programs could do more to ensure that new investigators of all backgrounds recognize the differences in health among racial and ethnic groups and that they are capable of addressing related questions in their research. In this regard, research training might be enhanced by drawing on recent developments in medical education. In addition to actively recruiting minority students, medical schools today are increasingly mindful that all their students must be prepared to treat patients from a wide variety of backgrounds. In fact, such training will become a mandatory component of the medical curriculum before the end of the 1999-2000 academic year, with the adoption of new accreditation standards requiring that medical school faculty and students "demonstrate an understanding of the manner in which people of diverse cultures and belief systems perceive health and illness and respond to various symptoms, diseases, and treatments."[11] The 1994 federal requirement that minority groups be adequately represented in clinical studies funded by the NIH and the Agency for Healthcare Research and Quality is another compelling reason for clinical research training programs to prepare trainees and fellows to work with diverse populations of patients.[12]

THE NATIONAL RESEARCH SERVICE AWARD PROGRAM AND OTHER FORMS OF RESEARCH TRAINING SUPPORT

In drafting the NRSA Act of 1974, Congress sought to strengthen the NIH's capacity to conduct research

---

[8] "MARC Undergraduate Student Training in Academic Research (U-STAR) Program," *NIH Guide for Grants and Contracts*, 29 July 1998. Available: http://grants.nih.gov/grants/guide/index/html.

[9] Ready, Timothy, and Herbert W. Nickens. Programs That Make a Difference. In *More Minorities in Health*, edited by Barbara H. Kehrer and Hugh Burroughs. Menlo Park, Calif.: The Henry J. Kaiser Foundation, 1994.

[10] Iler, Elisabeth, and Morton Slater. "The Gateway Program: Ten-Year Lessons About Outcomes and Admissions Measures." *Academic Medicine* 73, no. 11 (1998): 1169-71.

[11] Liaison Committee on Medical Education. "Accreditation Standards: Standards Proposed and Under Consideration." Online. Available: http://www. lcme.org/standard.htm. Accessed 8 December 1999.

[12] "NIH Guidelines on the Inclusion of Women and Minorities as Subjects in Clinical Research," *NIH Guide for Grants and Contracts*, 18 March 1994. Available: http://grants.nih.gov/grants/guide/index.html.

training by consolidating the agency's existing training activities into a single program. With the passage of this legislation, Congress expected that the NRSA program would become the "major element" of NIH training activities, providing a "consolidated authority in the Office of the Director of the National Institutes of Health [that] would enable resources to be flexibly adjusted each year to respond to the specific needs for the training of biomedical reseachers."[13]

In its early years, the NRSA program functioned much as Congress intended, but as other NIH funding mechanisms have come to be more widely employed for training and related activities, the relative influence and effectiveness of the NRSA program have waned. Instead of "the major element" of NIH research training, the NRSA program is now one of a number of such activities that the agency supports. As noted in Chapter 1, the NRSA program provided funding to 14,443 trainees and fellows in 1975, nearly 45 percent more than the NIH supported through graduate research assistantships, postdoctoral research appointments, and career development awards. That balance has long since been reversed: More than 30,000 graduate students, postdoctoral fellows, and young professionals were estimated to be supported by the agency through non-NRSA sources in 1997 (see Table 1-2), almost twice the number of NRSA trainees and fellows. As a result, the NRSA program no longer plays the decisive role it once did in NIH funding for health research training.

As the lead agency for NRSA research training, the NIH actively manages the program, setting policies and procedures, monitoring the number of training grant and fellowship awards, and assessing the career outcomes of its participants. Because the NIH does not oversee non-NRSA training-related awards in a similar fashion, the agency has little control over how many students and young investigators are supported with such funds, the type of training they receive, and the quality of their educational experience.

For some training-related activities, such as career development awards, the NIH establishes general guidelines; each of the agency's institutes determines for itself how many awards it will make, the salary it will pay, and the time commitment expected of its award recipients. For other types of funding, such as graduate research assistantships, there is less oversight. The NIH restricts the maximum compensation for graduate research assistants but sets few other guidelines. Furthermore, neither the agency nor its institutes limit the number of assistantships available. In fact, because the information management system shared by the NIH and the Agency for Healthcare Research and Quality is not set up to collect information on graduate research assistants—or, for that matter, postdoctoral research support personnel—the two agencies cannot determine the number of assistantships they provide. (The figures cited in this report and employed by the agencies are drawn from university reports of the numbers of graduate students and postdoctorates and their primary sources of support.)

With its range of funding mechanisms and uneven oversight, the current system of research training in the biomedical and behavioral sciences is far from being the consolidated flexible program that Congress envisioned. Our committee believes that research training in the health sciences is unlikely to meet national needs unless it is subject to greater oversight, consolidation, and control. Accomplishing this goal need not entail new legislation or a new research training program, but would require the NIH and other agencies to track training-related activities outside the NRSA program to manage the overall number of individuals trained in each field in response to research needs, and to coordinate a wider range of policies and procedures.

To better manage research training, the NIH, the Agency for Healthcare Quality and Research, and the Health Resources and Services Administration will require more detailed data on the research training activities they support. In particular, these agencies need better information on the number, characteristics, and compensation of students and postdoctorates supported by their research funds (including those working on the NIH campus), as well as on the training and research careers of physicians, dentists, and other health care professionals. Though data on NRSA participants are relatively complete, their fields of training are not consistently and accurately recorded, a gap in information that limits the agencies' ability to direct research training to areas of need.

Our committee was pleased to learn that the NIH is developing a new management information system (IMPAC II) and hopes the agency will take this opportunity to work with the Agency for Healthcare Research and Quality and the Health Resources and Services Administration to improve reporting on all research

[13] U.S. Congress. Senate Committee on Labor and Public Welfare. *National Research Service Award Act of 1974.* 93rd Cong., 1st sess., 1973. S. Rept. 93-381.

training and training-related activities, including fields of study. Future analyses of the research workforce would also be facilitated if the NIH's new management information system were routinely linked with other sources of data on the research workforce, such as the Doctorate Records File of Ph.D. recipients, the CRISP database of federally funded biomedical research projects, the Association of American Medical Colleges' Faculty Roster System, and the American Medical Association's Physician Masterfile.

In addition to improvements in data collection and analysis, the NIH, the Agency for Healthcare Research and Quality, and the Health Resources and Services Administration must pay additional attention to managing and coordinating their research training and related activities. Rather than relying solely on committees such as ours, which meet only periodically, the agencies should work together to bolster their capacity to analyze labor market trends on a continuing basis and to use these analyses to regulate the size and focus of their research training activities. Both research training and related activities should be guided by an explicit statement of educational philosophy, and the agencies should work together to coordinate policies and procedures, including those concerning stipends and eligibility for training, two issues that are discussed in greater detail below.

SETTING STIPENDS AND OTHER COMPENSATION

While pursuing NRSA research training, participating students and fellows receive stipends to help defray their living expenses. As shown in Table 5-2, stipend levels are determined by education and experience and rise as a student progresses from college to graduate school to postdoctoral training. At the postdoctoral level, stipends increase with every year of experience beyond the doctoral degree.

In contrast to NRSA participants, graduate students and postdoctorates who work as research assistants on federally funded research projects or on the NIH campus are regarded as employees. For part- or full-time work, these students and fellows receive salaries and other benefits, such as health insurance and tuition waivers. Compensation for these workers usually reflects their education and experience, but exceptions are frequently made. For example, NIH policy permits universities to compensate graduate student research assistants at the same level as first-year postdoctoral employees, as long as their total compensation (the combination of salary, tuition remission, and benefits) does not exceed $26,000.[14]

TABLE 5-2 NRSA Stipends, Fiscal Year 1999

Status	Stipend (in dollars)
Undergraduate students	
Freshmen/sophomores	6,780
Juniors/seniors	9,492
Graduate students	14,688
Postdoctorates (by years of experience)	
0	26,256
1	27,720
2	32,700
3	34,368
4	36,036
5	37,680
6	39,348
7 or more	41,268

SOURCE: "National Research Service Award (NRSA) Stipend Increase," *NIH Guide for Grants and Contracts*, 20 November 1998.

Though not every university provides the $26,000 maximum, compensation for graduate research assistants commonly exceeds the stipends and benefits provided to graduate students in NRSA training (see Table 2-1). For senior graduate students working on their dissertations, a higher level of compensation may well be appropriate to their advanced training and experience. Yet almost all universities also appoint first-year graduate students to research assistantships, a practice that can create disparities among entering students unless the institution subsidizes NRSA stipends to ensure that all students are compensated equally.

At the postdoctoral level, universities often synchronize salary levels with the NRSA stipend scale to ensure that postdoctoral fellows are treated equally throughout the institution. However, salaries for postdoctorates working on the NIH campus have routinely exceeded NRSA stipend levels, a discrepancy

[14] "Graduate Student Compensation," *NIH Guide for Grants and Contracts*, 2 December 1998. Available: http://grants.nih.gov/grants/guide/index.html.

that elicited complaints from university-based postdoctoral fellows. (Much of that disparity disappeared in 1998, when NRSA stipends increased approximately 25 percent.[15])

Because career development awards were originally designed for faculty members, salaries for these awards are higher than those granted to postdoctorates. Within limits set by each NIH institute, award recipients are compensated according to the salaries paid by their universities and research institutes. As a result, career development awards are the only training-related grants that recognize income differences among fields. Because of this flexibility, NIH staff have increasingly turned to career development awards in recent years as a means for providing research training to those in highly compensated fields such as bioinformatics and medicine.

By design, the NRSA program makes no distinctions between the stipends offered to M.D.s and Ph.D.s. When Congress established the program, its members were troubled by the then-common practice of providing higher stipends to M.D.s in research training than to Ph.D.s—especially since many physicians who undertook research training during that era did not eventually pursue research or academic careers. Thus, in establishing the NRSA program, Congress directed its administrators to eliminate the discrepancy between stipends provided to M.D.s and Ph.D.s.[16] Consequently, stipends for NRSA participants have always been determined by a single stipend scale.

While it is unlikely that the compensation and benefits that students and postdoctorates receive from various federal funding mechanisms can ever be completely standardized, NIH and its fellow agencies could do more to make their policies and practices consistent. The emphasis on education and experience that governs NRSA stipend levels should be applied to all training-related activities.

If, for example, the NIH believes that advanced graduate students should be compensated at higher levels than those just beginning their studies, that policy should apply throughout its training-related activities. Similarly, if the compensation for young professionals receiving career development awards recognizes salary differences among fields, the committee believes that the NIH and its fellow agencies should adopt the same approach for those in research training or training-related pursuits after the second or third postdoctoral year, when Ph.D.s have generally completed a postdoctoral fellowship and most M.D.s have completed their residency training.

On a related note, the committee was troubled that, although career development awards routinely cover family health insurance, the NRSA program provides only individual health insurance to participating graduate students and postdoctorates. The committee believes that the NIH, the Agency for Healthcare Research and Quality, and the Health Resources and Services Administration should require that family health insurance be provided to all eligible NRSA participants.

Finally, just as the NIH and the Agency for Healthcare Research and Quality research budgets are routinely adjusted every year for inflation, the same practice should be applied to the NRSA program and other training-related award mechanisms. Typically, NRSA stipends have been modified on an ad hoc basis, when the NIH budget permitted, and have not always kept up with inflation (see Figure 5-1). Moreover, because the higher levels apply only to training grants and fellowships awarded after the new stipend scale is in place, these intermittent adjustments can create significant discrepancies in the stipends paid to NRSA participants and between NRSA training programs and other training-related activities. The NIH, the Agency for Healthcare Quality and Research, and the Health Resources and Services Administration could do much to reduce these disparities if they modified their budgets annually to allow for increases in stipends, salaries, and other training-related costs and regularly adjusted compensation limits for career development awards.

THE TRAINING OF FOREIGN STUDENTS AND FELLOWS

Over the last few decades, steadily increasing numbers of foreign students and postdoctorates have sought research training in the health sciences at U.S. universities, medical centers, and research institutes. This trend has been most pronounced in the basic biomedical and clinical sciences but has been evident in the behavioral and social sciences as well (see Table 5-3). In the basic biomedical sciences, temporary-visa hold-

[15] "National Research Service Award (NRSA) Stipend Increase," *NIH Guide for Grants and Contracts*, 19 November 1998. Available at http://grants.nih.gov/grants/guide/index.html.

[16] U.S. Congress. Senate Committee on Labor and Public Welfare. *National Research Service Award Act of 1974.* 93rd Cong., 1st sess., 1973. S. Rept. 93-381.

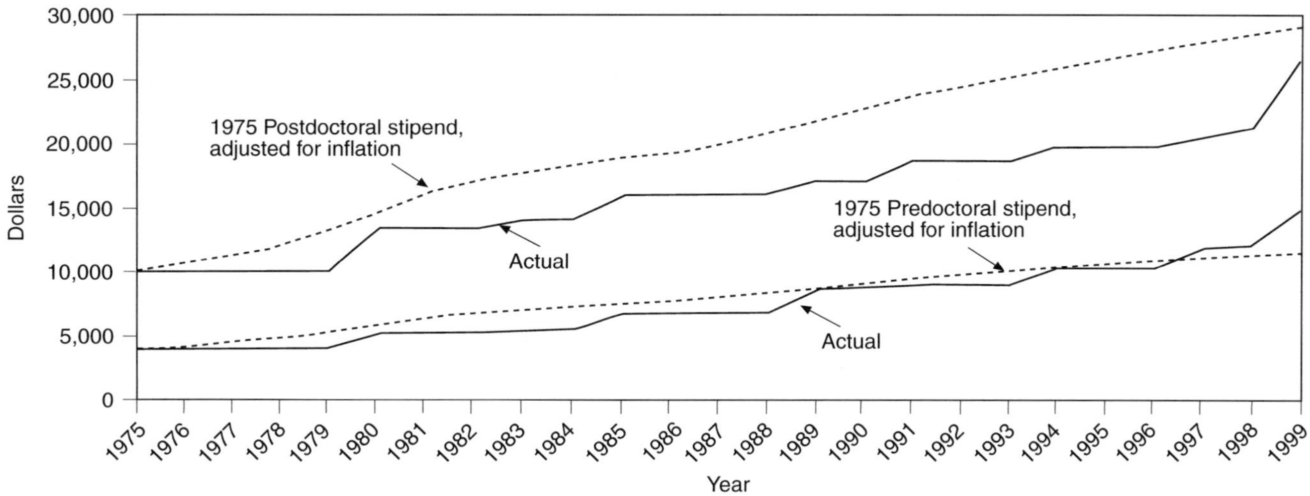

FIGURE 5-1 NRSA stipends for graduate students and first-year postdoctorates, actual and adjusted for inflation. SOURCE: Data are from the NIH Office of Extramural Research; adjustments were made using the Consumer Price Index.

ers account for more than 40 percent of the increase in the total number of Ph.D.s awarded since 1975.

Moreover, many of these temporary-visa holders who earn a Ph.D. in the U.S. remain in the country after completing their studies. After reviewing records from the Social Security Administration, one researcher found that 57 percent of Ph.D. recipients in the life sciences and 26 percent of Ph.D.s in the social sciences were still in the U.S. two years after receiving their doctorates.[17] Trends in the citizenship of postdoctoral fellows have not been tracked as long as for Ph.D. recipients, but from 1979 to 1997 the numbers of postdoctorates from other countries in the U.S. more than quadrupled in the biomedical and clinical sciences and more than tripled in the behavioral and social sciences. Altogether, biomedical, behavioral, and clinical departments of U.S. universities, medical schools, and research institutes reported hosting more than 12,500 foreign doctorates for training and employment in 1997—nearly 50 percent of postdoctorates in these three fields.[18]

Eligibility restrictions for most federal research training programs limit participation to U.S. citizens and permanent residents. As a result, NIH financial

[17] Finn, Michael G. "Stay Rates of Foreign Doctorate Recipients from U.S. Universities, 1995." Oak Ridge, Tenn.: Oak Ridge Institute for Science and Education, 1997.

[18] Unpublished tabulation from the Survey of Graduate Students and Postdoctorates in Science and Engineering; on file in the archives of the Academies.

TABLE 5-3 Ph.D.s Awarded to Temporary-Visa Holders

	1975			1997		
	No. of Temp.-Visa Holders	Total Ph.D.s	Percent	No. of Temp.-Visa Holders	Total Ph.D.s	Percent
Basic biomedical sciences	256	3,085	8.3	1,170	5,420	21.6
Behavioral and social sciences	190	2,794	6.8	253	2,591	9.8
Clinical sciences	21	230	9.1	247	1,349	18.3

SOURCE: Data are from the Survey of Earned Doctorates (see Tables G-1, G-2, and G-3).

support for foreign graduate students and postdoctorates is difficult to track, as their salaries and tuition benefits are most often included in budget lines for "research assistants" rather than for "training." The committee heard concerns that foreign graduate students and postdoctorates are seen by some American institutions as low-wage laboratory workers, rather than as young scientists undergoing intensive research training. Indeed, a number of American universities actively recruit foreign students for such purposes.[19] Such practices were defended by some on grounds of insufficient numbers of American-born and -educated biomedical scientists available to serve in research support roles.

Policies regarding the support of foreign students and postdoctorates vary considerably between the NRSA program and the other training-related activities of the NIH and AHRQ. For example, tuition waivers and other research training opportunities are available to graduate students and postdoctorates from anywhere in the world through federally-funded research projects at U.S. universities. At the same time, however, participation in NRSA training grants and fellowships is limited to U.S. citizens and permanent residents. The rationale for having these two different policies is not clear to the committee. If, for example, the reason for supporting foreign students and scientists on research grants is a rising demand for support staff to carry out research, rather than demand for principal investigators (as several recent reports have suggested),[20-22] federal policy-makers should turn their attention to developing a long-term solution to this need.

Federal officials should also review situations in which U.S. funds might reasonably be used to support the graduate education and postdoctoral research training of foreign citizens. The committee believes that federal funding of the educational expenses of foreign students and postdoctoral fellows should focus on foreign assistance programs intended to improve the scientific and technical personnel of developing countries and formal exchange programs, such as those currently sponsored by the NIH's Fogarty International Center. Whatever the final determinations of federal policymakers, the goal of federal funding for the education of foreign students and postdoctorates should be clearly articulated and funding should be tracked and managed to meet those objectives.

IMPLICATIONS AND RECOMMENDATIONS

When Congress established the NRSA program, it did so with the expectation that health research would benefit from a consolidated flexible program of research training. Yet over the years the NRSA program has had difficulty accommodating its system of predoctoral and postdoctoral training grants and fellowships to such challenges as the nation's increasing diversity, the growing demand for research support personnel, and the mounting indebtedness of health care professionals. As a result, research administrators and investigators have increasingly turned to funding mechanisms outside the NRSA program: research grant supplements and bridge grants for the training of underrepresented minorities, graduate research assistantships and postdoctoral appointments to fill the needs for research support staff, and career development awards for clinical investigator training.

These funding mechanisms appear to have filled some gaps in research training that the NRSA program was slow or unable to address. Even so, the resulting research workforce will not meet the nation's needs for health research unless these alternative funding mechanisms are thoughtfully coordinated with NRSA training grants and fellowships.

Recommendation 5-1. Led by NIH, the agencies with responsibility for health research training should strengthen their efforts to ensure diversity in the research workforce.

The NIH, the Agency for Healthcare Research and Quality, and the Health Resources and Services Administration should continue to evaluate existing programs intended to increase the diversity of the research workforce and redirect their funds, when appropriate, to programs and activities that have a measurable effect on diversity. The committee urges the agencies to focus their attention on improve-

---

[19] Burgess, David R."Barriers to Graduate School for Minority-Group Students." *Chronicle of Higher Education* 44, no. 7 (10 October 1997): B7-8.

[20] Massy, William F., and Charles A. Goldman. *The Production and Utilization of Science and Engineering Doctorates in the United States.* Stanford Institute for Higher Education Research Discussion Paper. Stanford, Calif.: 1995.

[21] National Research Council. *Trends in the Early Careers of Life Scientists.* Washington, D.C.: National Academy Press, 1998.

[22] Marincola, Elizabeth, and Frank Solomon. "The Career Structure in Biomedical Research: Implications for Training and Trainees." The American Society for Cell Biology Survey on the State of the Profession. *Molecular Biology of the Cell* 9 (November 1998), 3003-6.

ments in opportunities for minorities at the secondary school level (or earlier), seeking legislative authority to do so, if necessary. Though these agencies have not traditionally played much of a role in secondary education, we believe that their responsibility for ensuring diversity in the research workforce necessitates that they do so.

Recommendation 5-2. The NIH, the Agency for Healthcare Research and Quality, and the Health Resources and Services Administration should encourage research training programs to expose participants of all backgrounds to issues associated with economic, cultural, racial, and ethnic disparities in health.

While members of minority groups underrepresented in science may be more likely than others to be aware of the health problems of disadvantaged populations, they cannot and should not be expected to shoulder the responsibility for addressing the nation's needs for research in this arena. Research training should do more to ensure that greater numbers of investigators of all backgrounds are conscious of the differences in health among racial and ethnic groups and are capable of addressing related questions in their research.

Recommendation 5-3. The NIH, the Agency for Healthcare Research and Quality, and the Health Resources and Services Administration should consolidate their oversight of research training and training-related activities and thereby shape and manage the workforce as envisioned by Congress when it established the NRSA program.

We believe—just as Congress did when it authorized the NRSA program—that research training will be strengthened by more comprehensive oversight, consolidation, and control. In particular, there is a clear need for the NIH and the other agencies involved in the NRSA program to enhance their capacities to conduct regular analyses of labor market conditions affecting the research workforce.

Recommendation 5-4. Stipends and other forms of compensation for those in training should be based on education and experience and should be regularly adjusted to reflect changes in the cost of living.

While it is unlikely that the compensation and benefits that students and postdoctorates receive from various federal funding mechanisms can ever be completely standardized, the NIH, the Agency for Healthcare Research and Quality, and the Health Resources and Services Administration can do more to make their policies and practices consistent. The committee believes that the criteria of education and experience that determine NRSA stipend levels should guide compensation levels for training-related activities outside the NRSA program as well.

The committee welcomes the recent increases in NRSA stipends, yet notes that even the new stipend levels remain unduly low in view of the high levels of education and professional skills involved. The committee urges that automatic cost-of-living adjustments using appropriate indices be incorporated into budget planning, so that stipends are not again allowed to decline in real value.

Recommendation 5-5. The NIH and other federal science agencies that support research training should articulate clear goals regarding the education of foreign scientists and should modify their grants policies where necessary.

Policies regarding the support of foreign students and postdoctorates vary considerably between the NRSA program and the other training-related activities of the NIH and AHRQ. For example, tuition waivers and other research training opportunities are available to graduate students and postdoctorates from anywhere in the world through federally-funded research projects at U.S. universities. At the same time, however, participation in NRSA training grants and fellowships is limited to U.S. citizens and permanent residents. The rationale for having these two different policies is not clear to the committee. Federal goals for financing the education of foreign scientists should be more clearly defined and funding should be actively managed to meet those objectives.

Appendixes

Appendix A

National Research Service Award Institutional Training Grants and Fellowships

The National Research Service Award (NRSA) program supports research training at the predoctoral and postdoctoral levels. At each level awards may be made directly to individuals, who use the support at an institution of their choice, or to institutions, which in turn make awards to individuals. A brief description of the institutional training grant and fellowship awards included in the NRSA program can be found below.

INSTITUTIONAL AWARDS

Institutional Research Training Grants (T32)—Awarded to eligible institutions to develop or enhance predoctoral or postdoctoral research training opportunities for individuals, selected by the institution, who are training for careers in specified areas of biomedical and behavioral research. The Medical Scientist Training Program, which leads to the combined M.D.-Ph.D., and the Dental Scientist Training Program, which results in a D.D.S. or D.M.D. and Ph.D., are specialized institutional training grants.

Minority Access to Research Career (MARC) and Career Opportunities in Research (COR) Undergraduate Institutional Training Grants (T34)—Awarded to eligible institutions to support the undergraduate education of minority students to prepare them to compete successfully for entry into graduate programs leading to a Ph.D. degree in the biomedical or behavioral sciences.

Short-Term Institutional Research Training Grants (T35)—Awarded to selected institutions to expose students in health professional schools to research during summer breaks or to provide short-term predoctoral or postdoctoral research training in focused, often emerging, scientific areas.

INDIVIDUAL AWARDS

Individual Predoctoral Fellowships (F30)—To provide predoctoral training that leads to the combined M.D.-Ph.D. degree in preparation for research careers in mental health, alcohol abuse, alcoholism, and drug abuse.

Individual Predoctoral Fellowships for Minority Students and Students with Disabilities (F31)—To furnish eligible predoctoral students with supervised research training in health and health-related areas leading to a research degree (e.g., a Ph.D.).

Individual Postdoctoral Fellowships (F32)—To provide postdoctoral research training to individuals who have received a Ph.D., M.D., D.D.S., D.V.M., or equivalent degree to broaden their scientific background and further their potential for research in health-related areas.

Senior Postdoctoral Fellowships (F33)—To allow experienced scientists to make major changes in the direction of their research careers, broaden their scientific background, or acquire new research training.

Minority Access to Research Careers (MARC) Faculty Fellowships (F34)—To provide advanced research training to faculty members from institutions with a substantial enrollment of students from underrepresented minority groups.

Appendix B

Committee on National Needs for Biomedical and Behavioral Scientists

Howard Hiatt, M.D., chair, is professor of medicine at Harvard Medical School and senior physician at the Brigham and Women's Hospital. Former head of the Department of Medicine at Beth Israel Hospital, Boston, and former dean of the Harvard School of Public Health, Dr. Hiatt received his M.D. from Harvard University. He has been a member of the Institute of Medicine of since 1971 and is also a member of the Association of American Physicians, the American Academy of Arts and Sciences (where he is director of the Initiatives for Children Program), the American Society for Clinical Investigation, the American Society for Biochemistry and Molecular Biology, and the American Public Health Association. His research articles have appeared in the *Journal of Molecular Biology, Nature, Science*, *Journal of Biological Chemistry*, *Journal of Clinical Investigation*, *New England Journal of Medicine*, and the *Journal of the American Medical Association*. In addition, he has written for the lay press in areas of America's health care system, disease prevention, health services research, and health implications of the nuclear arms race.

Gail H. Cassell, Ph.D., is vice president of infectious diseases, drug discovery research, and clinical investigation, Eli Lilly and Company, Lilly Research Laboratories, in Indianapolis, Indiana. She is the former Charles H. McCauley professor and chairman of the Department of Microbiology at the University of Alabama Schools of Medicine and Dentistry at Birmingham. Under her leadership, the department ranked first in the nation in research funding from the National Institutes of Health. Dr. Cassell has been involved in the establishment of science policy and legislation related to biomedical research and public health. She is a recent past president of the American Society for Microbiology and currently serves as chairman of its Public and Scientific Affairs Board. A member of the Institute of Medicine, she has served as an advisor to the White House Office of Science and Technology Policy on infectious diseases and indirect costs of research. She has also served as a member of the NIH Director's Advisory Committee and the Advisory Council of the National Institute of Allergy and Infectious Diseases. Dr. Cassell's major research contribution to the field of microbiology in the recent past has been the establishment of *Ureaplasma urealyticum* as a significant cause of chorioamnionitis and disease in premature human infants. She has received several national research awards, has published over 300 articles and book chapters, and holds an honorary degree from the Thomas Jefferson University Medical College.

Janice G. Douglas, M.D., is professor of medicine and professor of physiology and biophysics at Case Western Reserve University School of Medicine. She is also director of the Hypertension Division and vice chairperson for academic affairs for the Department of Medicine. Dr. Douglas received her M.D. from Meharry Medical College in Nashville, Tennessee, and is a member of the American Society for Clinical Investigation, the Association for American Physicians, the Association for Academic Minority Physicians (of which she is a past president), the Central Society for Clinical Research, and the Institute of Medicine. She has served on the Board of Directors of the American Board of Internal Medicine and the Advisory Council of the National Heart, Lung, and Blood Institute. Dr. Douglas has authored a substantial number of medical publications and has been a member of editorial boards and publication committees for a number of medical journals, including the *Journal of Clinical Investigation*, *American Journal of Physiology*, *Circulation*, *Journal of Laboratory and Clinical Medicine*, and *Ethnicity and Disease*.

Richard B. Freeman, Ph.D., is the Ascherman Chair of Economics at Harvard University. He serves as faculty cochair of the Harvard University Trade Union Program and is director of the National Bureau of Economic Research's Program in Labor Studies. At the London School of Economics he is executive director of the Programme in Discontinuous Economics, a major program in economic analysis using neural nets and new data mining tools. Dr. Freeman received his Ph.D. from Harvard University. He is a member of the American Academy of Arts and Sciences and has served on several panels of the National Academy of Sciences, including High Risk Youth, Post Secondary Education and Training in the Workplace, Employment and Technical Change, and Demographic and Economic Impacts of Immigration. Professor Freeman has published over 250 articles and has written or edited 21 books, several of which have been translated into French, Spanish, Chinese, and Japanese.

Lee Goldman, M.D., is the Julius R. Krevans Distinguished Professor and chair of the Department of Medicine at the University of California, San Francisco, where he also serves as associate dean for clinical affairs in the School of Medicine. He received an M.D. and M.P.H. from Yale University School of Medicine and an honorary M.A. from Harvard University. His major research interests include the prediction of diagnosis and outcome of common cardiac complaints and problems, clinical utility and cost effectiveness of diagnostic tests and therapeutic interventions, and development and application of multivariate analytical techniques. Dr. Goldman is a member of the American Society for Clinical Investigation, an officer of the Association of American Physicians, past president of the Society of General Internal Medicine, a member of the Association of Professors of Medicine, a director of the American Board of Internal Medicine, a member of the Institute of Medicine, and a fellow of the American Association for the Advancement of Science. He has served as an associate editor of the *New England Journal of Medicine* and is now editor of the *American Journal of Medicine*, as well as lead coeditor of the *Cecil Textbook of Medicine*.

Leland H. Hartwell, Ph.D., is president and director of the Fred Hutchinson Cancer Research Center and a member of the Department of Genetics at the University of Washington. His research has emphasized the identification of genetic programs that control cell division and mating in the yeast, *Saccharomyces cerevisiae*. He received his Ph.D. from the Massachusetts Institute of Technology. An American Cancer Society research professor and member of the National Academy of Sciences, he is a recipient of the Eli Lilly Award in Microbiology and Immunology, General Motors Sloan Award, Hoffman LaRoche Mattia Award, Gairdner Foundation International Award, Brandeis University Rosensteil Award, Sloan-Kettering Cancer Center Katharine Berkan Judd Award, the Genetics Society of America Medal, MGH Warren Triennial Prize, Columbia University Horwitz Award, American Society of Cell Biology's Keith Porter Award, Passano Award, and the Carnegie Mellon Dickson Prize.

John F. Kihlstrom, Ph.D., is professor of psychology at the University of California, Berkeley. He received his Ph.D. from the University of Pennsylvania and has previously served on the faculties of Harvard University, Stanford University, University of Wisconsin, University of Arizona, and Yale University. His research focuses on cognition in personality and social interaction, unconscious mental processes, and memory and has been funded continuously by the NIH since 1977. Dr. Kihlstrom currently holds a MERIT award from the National Institute of Mental Health. From 1992 to 1995 he served as cochair of the NIMH Basic Behavioral Science Task Force. He is a fellow of the American Association for the Advancement of Science, the American Psychological Association, and the Society for Clinical and Experimental Hypnosis and is a charter fellow of the American Psychological Society. Dr. Kihlstrom has published over 160 articles and book chapters, coauthored one book, and coedited three others. Additionally, he has held a number of editorial appointments and currently serves as the editor of *Psychological Science*.

Ellen M. Markman, Ph.D., is associate dean for the social sciences and professor of psychology at Stanford University. She received her Ph.D. from the University of Pennsylvania. Her research interests are cognitive and early language development. Dr. Markman has been a member of the Advisory Board of *Learning,*

Development, and Conceptual Change (Bradford Books), the Cognition, Emotion, and Personality Review section in NIMH, the Child Development Subcommittee of the Social Science Research Council, the Steering Committee of the Study of Stanford and the Schools, the Executive Committee of the Sloan Cognitive Science Program at Stanford (which she also chaired), the Governing Council of the Society for Research in Child Development, and the Executive Committee of the Children and Society Curriculum. She has served on a number of editorial boards, including those for *Cognitive Psychology*, *Cognitive Development*, *Contemporary Psychology*, *Developmental Psychology*, and *Child Development*. Dr. Markman is the author of one book and over 50 articles that have appeared in *Corrective Psychiatry, Child Development, Cognition, Contemporary Psychology, Cognitive Psychology, Developmental Psychology, Journal of Educational Psychology, Merrill Palmer Quarterly*, and *American Scientist*, among others.

Edward E. Penhoet, Ph.D., is dean of the School of Public Health, University of California, Berkeley. He is former president and chief executive officer of the Chiron Corporation in Emeryville, California, and now serves as adjunct professor of molecular and cell biology at the University of California, Berkeley. He received his Ph.D. in biochemistry from the University of Washington. Dr. Penhoet is a member of the American Society of Biological Chemists, the American Association for the Advancement of Science, and the American Chemical Society. He is the author of over 50 articles that have appeared in the *Proceedings of the National Academy of Sciences*, *Annals New York Academy of Science*, *Biochemistry*, *Federation Proceedings*, *Journal of Biological Chemistry*, *Journal of Virology, Journal of the National Cancer Institute, Methods in Enzymology, Developmental Biology, Molecular Biology and Medicine*, and the *American Journal of Human Genetics*, among others.

Steven A. Schroeder, M.D., is president of the Robert Wood Johnson Foundation in Princeton, New Jersey. He also practices general internal medicine part-time at the Robert Wood Johnson Medical School, where he is clinical professor of medicine. He received his M.D. from Harvard Medical School and honorary doctorates from Rush University, Boston University, and the University of Massachusetts. Dr. Schroeder has been a member of many health care organizations, including Alpha Omega Alpha, the American College of Physicians (master), the American Public Health Association, the Association of American Physicians, the Institute of Medicine, the United States Prospective Payment Assessment Commission, and the Society of General Internal Medicine (of which he is a past president). He chairs the International Advisory Committee of the Faculty of Medicine at Ben-Gurion University in Israel. To his credit are more than 200 publications in the fields of clinical medicine, health care organization and financing, manpower, quality of care, and preventive medicine. He has served on a number of editorial boards, including, at present, the *New England Journal of Medicine*.

Michael S. Teitelbaum, D. Phil., is a program director at the Alfred P. Sloan Foundation in New York, New York. He received his D.Phil. in demography from Oxford University, where he was a Rhodes scholar, and has been a member of the faculties of Oxford University and Princeton University, staff director of the Select Committee on Population in the U.S. House of Representatives, and a professional staff member of the Ford Foundation and of the Carnegie Endowment for International Peace. He has also served as a commissioner of the U.S. Commission for the Study of International Migration and Cooperative Economic Development. He was elected first vice president of the Population Association of America, the scientific society of demographers, and until December 1997 was vice chair of the U.S. Commission on Immigration Reform. Dr. Teitelbaum is a regular speaker on demographic change, immigration, and the science and engineering workforce, and a frequently invited witness before committees of the U.S. Congress and publishes extensively in scientific and popular journals and in national op-ed pages. He is the author of five books and many articles.

Appendix C

Public Comment on the National Research Service Award Program

To gain a better understanding of the conditions and forces that affect training needs, the Committee on National Needs for Biomedical and Behavioral Scientists solicited public comment from experts in the fields supported by the National Research Service Award (NRSA) program. In letters to 885 investigators, directors of training programs, graduate deans, representatives of industry, students, and postdoctoral fellows, the committee posed questions such as the following:

- What role do NRSA traineeships and fellowships play in training for careers in biomedical, behavioral, and clinical research? How does the NRSA program compare in this regard with other forms of federal support, such as research assistantships, dissertation grants, and career development awards?
- What improvement should be made to NRSA traineeships and fellowships and to other forms of federal research training support?
- Should opportunities for research training be modified in response to (1) the expansion or contraction of particular research fields or (2) trends in the hiring of researchers by universities, industry, and academic health centers? If so, how?

The committee received 109 responses to its inquiry, which are summarized below.

THE ROLE OF THE PROGRAM

Many respondents regarded the NRSA program as the single most important component in the continuum of research training support in the biomedical and behavioral sciences and described the program as "invaluable," "critical," "irreplaceable," and "essential." Others noted that "these programs feed the whole research engine of this country" and that they "set the gold standard for quality students, faculty, and programmatic aspects of graduate education." Several present or former award recipients reported that they would not have been able to attend graduate school or would not have succeeded in their careers without NRSA support.

Other funding mechanisms for research training in the basic biomedical and behavioral and social sciences complement the NRSA program but do not generally compete with it. NRSA traineeships and fellowships are generally offered to those in the early phases of pre- or postdoctoral study. Research assistantships and dissertation grants, on the other hand, are often reserved for students at more advanced stages of study and emphasize the applications of skills to a specific research project, rather than to the development of a broad base of knowledge. Graduate students from other countries, however, are an exception to this rule. Because they are not eligible for NRSA support, foreign students may be appointed to research assistantships from the time they enter graduate school.

Less research-intensive institutions, where research assistantships are not as readily available, report that they depend heavily on NRSA support. Much the same appears to be the case in such fields as clinical research, where research assistantships are not as common as in the basic biomedical sciences. For prospective clinical investigators, the NRSA program may be the primary source or one of only a few sources of research training support.

The NRSA program offers benefits beyond financial support for its participants. Predoctoral awardees usually complete their degrees more quickly than their classmates who do not have NRSA support, because this funding allows them to concentrate on their studies, rather than on teaching duties or their mentor's research.

NRSA fellowship holders, whether at the pre- or postdoctoral level, are provided a level of independence not generally experienced with other mechanisms of support. Applicants for fellowships choose their own mentors and projects, and those who ultimately receive awards have greater control over their time than do their counterparts who work on research grants. Applying for a fellowship, furthermore, provides students and postdoctorates the opportunity to gain experience in preparing a proposal and to become familiar with the application process itself—an important preview of life as an independent investigator.

On the whole, respondents believed that the NRSA program provides its participants with a good start on a research career. As one letter writer reported, "We can place trainees in the very best postgraduate programs or faculty positions." Another maintained that most trainees go into academic research careers and that NRSA recipients in clinical fields often stayed in research, even if only part-time.

Beyond the direct effect on funding recipients, the NRSA program is widely thought to enhance the overall quality of training in the biomedical and behavioral sciences. The requirement for instruction in the responsible conduct of research, for example, often prompts institutions to provide ethics training to all students. Likewise, training grants may provide funds for retreats, seminars, and other activities that benefit all students and contribute to creating a "community of scholars." The prospect of competing for training grants and fellowships, furthermore, motivates all applicants to strive for excellence, even if they do not obtain an award.

PROGRAM IMPROVEMENTS

While respondents praised the NRSA program on the whole, they also had suggestions for improvement, most of which centered on program funding. The most common recommendation was that stipends be increased. [Note: In November of 1998, following the completion of the public comment process, the National Institutes of Health, the Agency for Healthcare Research and Quality, and the Health Resources and Services Administration announced that stipends for NRSA awards made in fiscal year 1999 would increase by approximately 25 percent for trainees and fellows at all levels of experience.] Respondents also suggested that the number of trainees and fellows be expanded, that the length of awards be increased, and that funding for various aspects of the program (e.g., health insurance and tuition) be improved.

In making the case for a stipend increase, respondents often cited the other research training options and career paths available to students and fellows. Outside the NRSA program, graduate students receive higher stipends with a National Science Foundation Graduate Research Fellowship and may earn more and receive greater benefits working as a research assistant. One respondent noted that students in his department generally prefer research assistantships to NRSA funding because their compensation as a research assistant is higher.

At the postdoctoral level, one respondent called for stipends to be increased to the level of salaries for postdoctorates working on the National Institutes of Health (NIH) campus. Others recommended that stipends for health care professionals should be comparable to what M.D.s earn as residents, for example, or what nurses earn in practice. In addition to increased stipends, a number of respondents suggested loan forgiveness for physicians and dentists, so that they would not feel compelled to forgo a research career in order to pay back their educational debt.

A number of respondents called for stipends to be indexed to inflation or the cost of living in a particular area. One writer complained that stipends were too low to support someone living in Los Angeles; another made the same observation about the difference between the stipends and the cost of living in New York City.

The comments about educational payments for NRSA trainees and fellows echoed those made about stipends: They should be increased. Most respondents believed that NRSA reimbursement for tuition is too low, which forces institutions to accept significant cost sharing. On this point, however, there was less consensus than on the subject of stipends. A few commentators suggested that universities have a responsibility to support some tuition costs or even waive tuition for NRSA recipients.

In addition to increasing stipends and tuition reimbursement, another common suggestion was to increase the number of participants and extend the length of their tenure. In particular, some thought that training grants and fellowships should be granted to a wider range of institutions than at present. While NRSA policy allows for five years of predoctoral support, some NIH institutes encourage universities to limit appointments on NRSA training grants to three years or less; many respondents thought this practice was unrealistic, as it generally takes seven years to complete a Ph.D. in the biomedical sciences. Other respondents raised similar concerns about the policy limiting postdoctoral awards to three years. One letter writer suggested that bridge awards be established to fill the gap between the end of an NRSA postdoctoral appointment and eligibility for other awards.

Regarding other aspects of the program, many commentators called for increased funding for health insurance, equipment, travel, and administration. One postdoctoral fellow lamented that after paying his health insurance premium, little money was left for research supplies. Noting the heavy administrative workload that accompanies a training grant, one respondent suggested such awards include support for a portion of the director's salary. Another recommended that training grants include funds for at least a part-time administrative assistant.

Beyond suggestions for improved funding, a number of respondents called for expanded eligibility for research training support. Some commentators believed that foreign nationals, particularly those who are applying for permanent residency, should be permitted to participate in NRSA programs. Others were concerned that the requirement for full-time research training discourages the recruitment and retention of women and recommended that part-time research training be an option.

Finally, some respondents expressed dissatisfaction with the length and cumbersome nature of the review process. Their recommendations for improvement included simplifying application forms and reducing the time required for review.

SUGGESTED MODIFICATIONS IN RESPONSE TO WORKFORCE TRENDS

Respondents were resoundingly opposed to reducing the overall size of the NRSA program. If additional funds become available, they believe that it merits expansion.

There was much less consensus on the question of whether research training in specific fields should be modified in response to hiring patterns or the expansion or contraction of research opportunities, but the majority of the respondents believed that "careful" adjustments could be beneficial. Some called for a modification in research training in fields where there are few academic positions available, with one individual noting that overtraining wastes resources and denies training opportunities to others. Respondents disagreed about whether the NIH or local mentors should be responsible for making the necessary decisions, but a number believed that the process should be guided by periodic program reviews. One person recommended a survey of prospective employers.

Of the fields singled out for increases in research training, the ones mentioned most often were generally in the clinical and behavioral sciences, such as health services research, outcomes research, nursing, dentistry, and epidemiology and biostatistics. Also mentioned were bioinformatics and a wide variety of clinical and behavioral research fields. Other commentators suggested an increase in broad-based, interdisciplinary research training programs to help prospective investigators respond to future research advances.

Most respondents did not consider whether increases in research training support might result in cuts in other forms of funding. Of those that did, most would shift support from research assistantships to training grants; within the NRSA program others suggested reallocating funds from individual fellowships to training grants.

The very few fields that were singled out for reductions in research training included gastroenterology, veterinary science, and nursing.

Many respondents made suggestions about the evaluation—and reevaluation—of research training programs, so as to establish which are the most successful and which should be expanded or contracted. Several commentators recommended that the outcomes of training grants and fellowship awards be compared to determine where additional funds should be directed.

Appendix D

Demographic Projections of the Ph.D. Workforce in Biomedical and Behavioral Research, 1995-2005

The growth of any workforce is always subject to unexpected change—to new technologies, new market conditions, and changing national needs. One can, however, make provisional projections if the current workforce can be accurately defined and if acceptable assumptions can be made about the entry of new workers into the field and their propensity to change fields, retire, or die. Using the best available data and what seem to be reasonable assumptions, such projections are made here over the period 1995-2005 for two major groups in the health research workforce: Ph.D.s in the basic biomedical and the behavioral and social sciences. Because of limited data, the projections do not include Ph.D.s in the clinical sciences or health care professionals in any field of health-related research. The assumptions used in projecting the workforce are essentially demographic. That is, they rely on historical tendencies of workers grouped by age and sex to enter, remain in, and leave the biomedical and behavioral workforce. Whether workers will act in accordance with such tendencies will of course be heavily affected by the job market, but the demand for labor is not directly modeled in this exercise.

The Ph.D. workforce in both biomedical and behavioral research has grown steadily over several decades, and projections show they will continue to grow from 1995 to 2005, though at varying rates: 3.4 percent annually in biomedical research and 1.2 percent in behavioral research. Growth in each field is projected to be greater among females than males, so that, by 2005, the number of females in biomedical research will reach about half the number of males, while females in behavioral research will about equal the number of males. The workforce will continue to grow older in each field, an inevitable result of slower workforce growth and longer times to degree, particularly in the behavioral sciences. By 2005 the median age among biomedical scientists is projected to have increased from 45.3 years to 46.2 years, and the median age among behavioral scientists will have risen more substantially from 48.8 years to 52.4 years.

These projections rely on a variety of assumptions: trends in the numbers of Ph.D. graduates extrapolated from previous trends, retirement schedules and rates for moving in and out of employment, and continued substantial shifts between science and nonscience jobs, especially among relatively younger Ph.D.s. Reasonable alternative assumptions about trends in graduates and immigrant Ph.D.s do not alter the projections substantially.

Simulations were run to determine the number of graduates required to maintain a constant workforce. In each field the required graduates would be substantially below current numbers. If, instead, the workforce were constrained to grow in parallel with the U.S. workforce as a whole, the number of graduates in behavioral and social research would decline initially and then recover. In basic biomedical fields, on the other hand, the number of graduates would be substantially smaller than current numbers.

BACKGROUND AND ASSUMPTIONS

The Potential Workforce

By definition, the basic biomedical sciences include biological science fields from anatomy to zoology (excluding the plant sciences), as well as the related fields of veterinary medicine, biomedical engineering, and pharmaceutical chemistry. Other life sciences are generally excluded but may be included in tabulations of graduate students because of differences in the design of the national surveys of graduate students and Ph.D.s. The behavioral and social sciences of interest include psychology, sociology, anthropology, demography, and speech-language pathology and audiology. Because this study focuses on research scientists, clinical, counseling, and school psychologists, who constitute more than 40 percent of recent Ph.D. graduates in these disciplines combined, are excluded in most tabulations.

The potential research workforce in the targeted fields is defined to include Ph.D.s who are either (1) employed full- or part-time in science or engineering, (2) unemployed but seeking work, or (3) not employed and not seeking work but not retired. Employment includes postdoctoral appointments. Because of data limitations, biomedical and behavioral Ph.D.s are included even if they are working in other scientific or engineering fields. Similar data limitations also result in the exclusion of Ph.D.s with degrees in other fields who have chosen to work in biomedical or behavioral sciences.

Those not employed and not seeking work are usually considered not to be in the labor force (and will be labeled as such). Among Ph.D.s in these fields, this group is overwhelmingly female. They move in and out of employment, and with the proportion of female Ph.D.s increasing, those not in the labor force are important to track as a potential source of trained labor. (The inclusion of this group is also the reason for using the somewhat unconventional label "potential workforce.")

People are assumed to enter the potential workforce when they (1) graduate with a Ph.D. in the biomedical or behavioral sciences and stay in the U.S., (2) immigrate to the U.S. after earning a Ph.D. abroad in these fields, or (3) shift from a job outside science to a job in science. The third category includes the few shifts from jobs outside science to unemployment or out of the labor force. Some additional possibilities that also involve small numbers of people will be ignored: return from retirement and, for U.S.-trained Ph.D.s. working abroad, return migration. (Excluding a return from retirement is one reason for distinguishing the retired from those not in the labor force, a number of whom return to employment.)

People are assumed to leave the potential workforce if they (1) take employment outside science, (2) retire, or (3) die. They may also emigrate, but data on emigrants are inadequate for analysis.

Figure D-1 illustrates the different groups and potential movements among them. Only the potential workforce itself and its three components—the employed, the unemployed, and those not in the labor force—will be projected, though for this purpose movement into and out of other groups has to be tracked.

Data

Survey data provide a picture of the potential workforce and show how it has evolved and thus permit parameters to be selected for the above model based on recent history. One source is the Survey of Doctorate Recipients, a longitudinal biennial survey dating

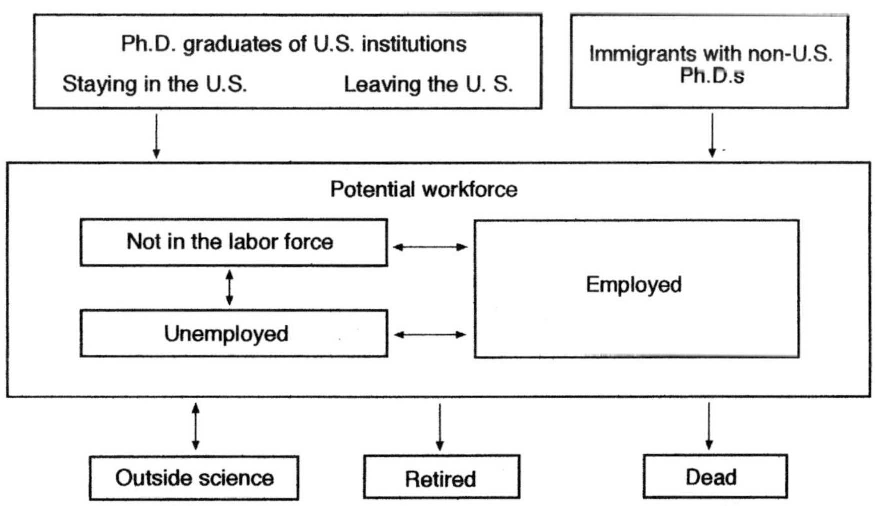

FIGURE D-1 The potential Ph.D. workforce of biomedical and behavioral scientists.

back to 1973. From 1973 to 1989, the universe for this survey included all Ph.D.s with degrees earned in the U.S. who planned to stay in the country, plus Ph.D.s with degrees from abroad who were employed in the U.S. prior to 1973 and received their doctorates no more than 42 years prior to the survey year. In 1991 the latter group was dropped, and an age limitation of 75 years was imposed.[1]

Ph.D. graduates entering the workforce are reported by the Survey of Earned Doctorates, a census conducted annually since 1920, with all results kept in a virtually complete database of research doctorates called the Doctorate Records File. Annual reports on the survey have been issued since 1967.[2]

Graduate enrollees and current enrollment were obtained from the Survey of Graduate Students and Postdoctorates in Science and Engineering.[3] This survey of graduate institutions provides a time series for current enrollment from 1979. Some data are available before 1979 but are irregular; in some years they are missing altogether and in others they fail to distinguish males from females. The survey also began to report numbers of first-time, full-time enrollees by field in 1980 but did not distinguish between clinical and nonclinical graduate students in psychology until 1988.

[1] National Science Foundation. *Characteristics of Doctoral Scientists and Engineers in the U.S.: 1991*. Arlington, Va.: NSF, 1994.

[2] National Research Council. *Summary Report 1996: Doctorate Recipients from U.S. Universities*. Washington, D.C.: National Academy Press, 1998.

[3] National Science Foundation. *Graduate Students and Postdoctorates in Science and Engineering: Fall 1997*. Arlington, Va.: NSF, 1999.

Immigration information was obtained from the 1993 and 1995 Surveys of College Graduates, which followed up a sample of postsecondary degree holders from the 1990 U.S. census.[4] These surveys, as well as the Survey of Doctorate Recipients, use a weighted sample. Weighted numbers that represent the population will be reported throughout; these numbers do not represent actual respondents. Respondents are often fewer, especially for immigrants, and particular figures cited may not have much precision. Where possible, data are aggregated to minimize this problem.

Data were also obtained on mortality from TIAA/CREF, the primary pension system for individuals employed in education and research.

Some analysis and interpretation of these data will be necessary, but this is not the main purpose of this exercise. For more information on the characteristics of and past trends in the workforce, a variety of other studies are available, such as *Trends in the Early Careers of Life Scientists*.[5]

The Current Workforce

The current potential workforce, which serves as the base for the projection, consists of 83,000 biomedical research Ph.D.s and 52,300 behavioral research Ph.D.s, according to the 1995 Survey of Doctorate Recipients (see Table D-1). Not counted in these figures are those

[4] National Science Foundation. *SESTAT: A Tool for Studying Scientists and Engineers in the U.S.* Arlington, Va.: NSF, 1999.

[5] National Research Council. *Trends in the Early Careers of Life Scientists*. Washington, D.C.: National Academy Press, 1998.

TABLE D-1 Ph.D. Workforce by Employment Status, Plus Those Outside Science and Retired, by Major Field and Gender, 1995

	Biomedical Ph.D.s		Behavioral Ph.D.s	
Employment Status	Male	Female	Male	Female
Employed	57,968	21,009	30,318	20,061
Unemployed	823	414	175	256
Not in labor force	1,097	1,672	466	1,048
Total potential workforce	59,888	23,095	30,959	21,365
Outside science	5,087	2,745	5,147	3,519
Retired	5,535	1,091	3,889	1,024

NOTE: The workforce is defined to exclude those outside of science and retired. Figures also exclude those over age 75.

SOURCE: Datra are from the Survey of Doctorate Recipients.

employed outside science, who are more numerous among behavioral researchers (8,700) than among biomedical researchers (7,800). Also not counted are Ph.D.s who obtained their degrees outside the U.S., a group that will be considered below.

Women make up 28 percent of the workforce in biomedical research and 41 percent in behavioral research. Most of the workforce—91 percent to 98 percent across broad fields and gender—is employed. Of the small proportions unemployed or not in the labor force, more than half in biomedical research and two-thirds in behavioral research are women.

The workforce in biomedical research is younger: 34 percent are 40 years old or younger, as opposed to 19 percent in behavioral research. Only 30 percent in biomedical research are over 50 years old, as opposed to 40 percent in behavioral research (see Figure D-2). Median ages are 46.5 years among male biomedical scientists, 42.4 years among females, 50.2 years among male behavioral scientists, 46.7 years among females. Since it is slightly older, the workforce in behavioral research could see proportionally more retirements and deaths over the next few decades than the workforce in biomedical research. Since men in both fields are somewhat older, retirements and deaths could contribute to a gradually rising proportion of women in each field.

Among those employed, 3.5 percent in the biomedical workforce and 7 percent in the behavioral workforce are employed less than full-time. The majority of part-time employees in both fields—75 percent—are not seeking full-time work, which suggests that most part-time employment is voluntary. Close to half the individuals working part-time in biomedical research and two-thirds of those in behavioral research are women. Part-time employment among women tends to be concentrated among those age 33-50, whereas part-time employment among men is substantially more common beyond age 60 than among younger men. Trends in part-time employment will not be projected but should be kept in mind. The distribution suggests relatively little possibility for increasing the output of biomedical and behavioral scientists by enticing part-time workers to work full-time.

Entry of New Graduates

Ph.D. graduates in 1995 totaled 5,100 in biomedical research and 2,400 in behavioral research, the equiva-

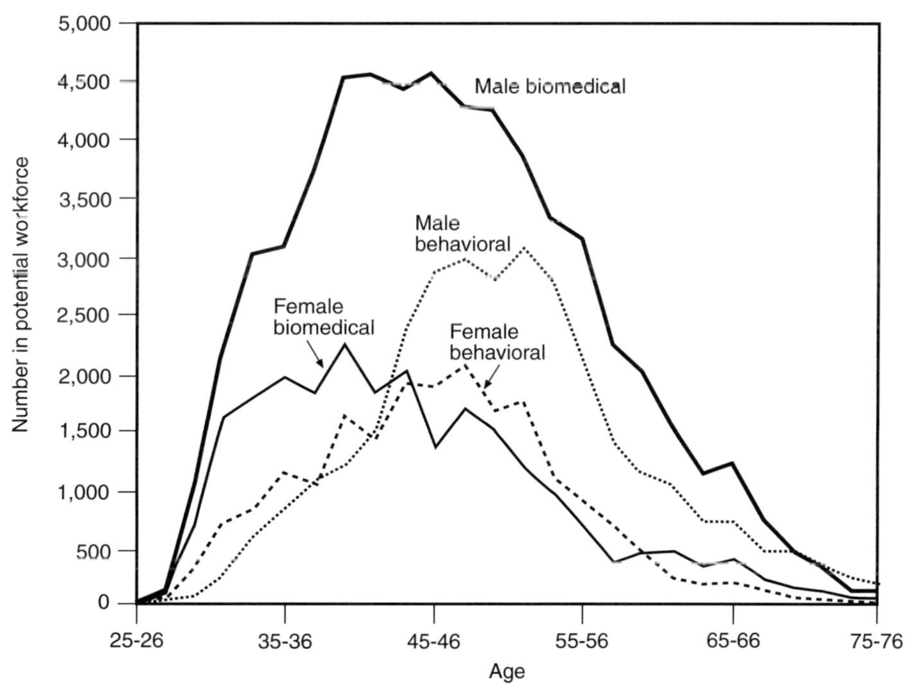

FIGURE D-2 Age distribution of potential workforce in 1995 by field and gender (in two-year age groups). SOURCE: Data are from the Survey of Doctorate Recipients.

lent of 6 percent and 4.5 percent of the potential workforce in the respective fields (though not all of the graduates may have entered the workforce).

The number of Ph.D. recipients in a given year may be expected to depend on the number of students who enrolled in graduate school six to nine years earlier, the time it usually takes to complete the requirements for a Ph.D. The ratio of entering graduate students to Ph.D. recipients six years later, however, is not stable but varies by field and gender as well as over time. This ratio has been as low as 1.4 enrollees per graduate (e.g., for 1990 male biomedical research enrollees) and as high of 2.8 enrollees per graduate (e.g., for 1990 female behavioral research enrollees). Regression analysis confirmed the lack of consistent linkage. When first-year enrollment rose, the number of graduates six to nine years later decreased at least as often as it increased. Regressions based on the total population of graduate students were no more successful. Only when a short time lag was used could one year's pool of students be used to predict the number of graduates in the next year or two.

The lack of a clear relationship between graduate school enrollment and Ph.D. production may be due partly to data limitations and the nature of graduate education itself. To begin with, counts of new students entering graduate school include those seeking master's as well as doctoral degrees. Even among those intending to earn a doctoral degree, time to degree is variable, and the six- to nine-year period allows students many opportunities to drop out. These limitations aside, there is a tendency for the numbers of Ph.D. recipients to rise a year or two after enrollment rises, which suggests that short-term job market conditions may lead to almost simultaneous increases in new enrollees, graduate students, and graduates. In a large pool of students, such economic factors may strongly influence some to finally earn or postpone earning their Ph.D.s in a given period.

The number of graduates therefore can be projected from reported enrollees or current students only for a year or possibly two. An alternative method projects graduates directly on the basis of historical trends (observable for a longer period), recognizing that such curve fitting is at least partly arbitrary. These trends can be quickly summarized. Since the 1960s, graduates have increased in both fields (see Figure D-3). After the early 1970s, however, male graduates in biomedical research remained largely constant for almost two decades before increasing recently, and male graduates in behavioral research declined. Female graduates in both fields have continued to increase.

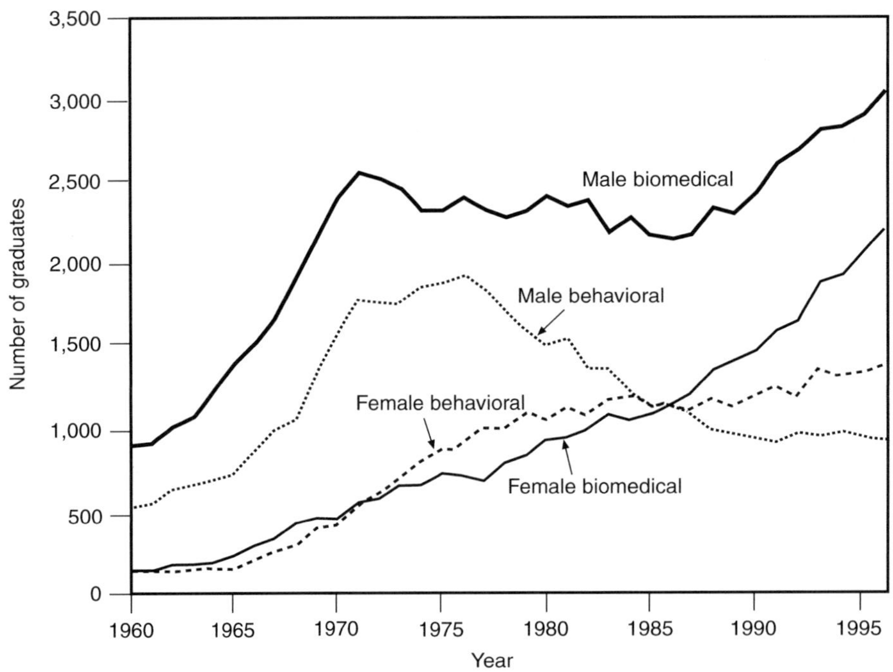

FIGURE D-3 New Ph.D. graduates by field and gender, 1960-96. SOURCE: Data are from the Survey of Earned Doctorates.

Projections based on these past trends vary depending on the period from which one extrapolates. Alternative periods were chosen—1970-96, 1975-96, and 1985-96—and trends were quantified using regression analysis. The regressions were for new graduates by field and gender, predicted from calendar year and year squared. These regressions generally fit the data well, with all R^2s being above 0.80. The regressions for 1985-96 typically showed the fastest rates of increase. None of the regressions for biomedical research indicated future declines in graduates, but for behavioral research the regressions for 1970-96 did suggest future declines (see the Technical Note later in this appendix).

For current purposes, the regressions for 1985-96 can be taken to define one possible set of scenarios for future graduates. The number of graduates increases in each group every year, in these scenarios, by 2 percent to 6 percent, faster than in trends extrapolated from other regressions. These may, therefore, be considered "high-growth" scenarios. An alternative "low-growth" scenario, for behavioral research graduates, may be the declining-graduates regressions based on 1970-96 data. For biomedical research graduates, simply keeping the numbers constant at average levels for 1990-96 will be used to produce a low scenario. In each case, a "medium-growth" scenario will be simply the average of the high and the low scenarios.

Some proportion of graduates, particularly non-U.S. citizens with temporary visas, will not stay in the country after graduation. The first issue is the number of graduates on temporary visas. By 1996, noncitizens had risen to 37 percent of biomedical research graduates and 16 percent of behavioral research graduates. About two-thirds of these were on temporary visas. The proportion of graduates on temporary visas almost doubled from 1985 to 1990, but from then on it fluctuated with no apparent pattern, while the proportion on permanent visas was increasing rapidly (see Figure D-4). The Chinese Student Protection Act of 1992 (which provided Chinese students with protection from political turmoil at home by allowing them to apply for permanent U.S. residency) had some influence on trends during the 1990s.[6] As a result of the law, the percentage of students from China who were permanent U.S. residents at the time they received their degree increased from 5

[6] National Research Council. *Summary Report 1995: Doctorate Recipients from U.S. Universities.* Washington, D.C.: National Academy Press, 1996.

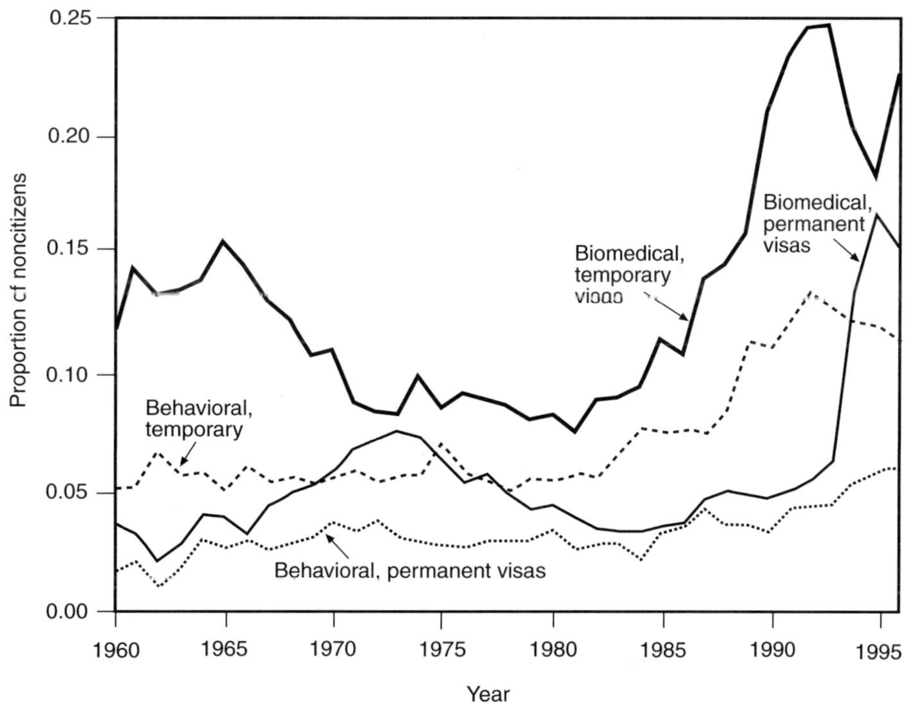

FIGURE D-4 Proportion of noncitizens among U.S. Ph.D. graduates by field and visa type, 1960-96. SOURCE: Data are from the Survey of Earned Doctorates

percent in 1990 to 80 percent in 1995. Extrapolating from these trends would, therefore, be unwise. Instead, for projection purposes, the proportion of temporary visas will be assumed to stay at its 1990-96 average for each group defined by field and sex. This means that those on temporary visas will be projected at 24 percent among male biomedical research graduates, 18 percent among females, 16 percent among male behavioral research graduates, and 9 percent among females.

The proportion of those on temporary visas that stay in the U.S. also appears to be rising, but these data are more difficult to obtain. By identifying Ph.D. graduates who later show up in Social Security Administration data, Finn[7] estimated that 60 percent of 1993 noncitizen graduates in the life sciences were still in the U.S. in 1995. The life sciences are somewhat broader than the biomedical sciences, for they also include agricultural sciences and basic biological sciences. A parallel estimate for 1993 graduates in the social sciences more broadly defined (including, besides those listed above, economics and urban and regional planning) was 35 percent. These proportions could be rising, given that equivalent estimates for the 1990-91 cohort in each field were 40 percent and 28 percent, respectively. As cohorts age, the numbers of foreign graduates still in the U.S. do not appear to fall—over five years or so, they may actually rise as Ph.D.s return from abroad. In the absence of more definitive evidence, however, the estimates for the 1993 cohort will be adopted here for both males and females for the projection period. All other graduates, citizens as well as noncitizens on permanent visas, will be projected to stay in the U.S.

Ph.D. graduates in these fields are most often in the age range of 30-34 years but may be as young as 25 years or over 45 years. The proportion age 25-29 years rose sharply from the 1960s to the 1970s and then declined while the proportion older than 29 years was rising. Greater delays in obtaining bachelor's degrees, delays in enrollment in graduate school, and increases in the time required to earn a Ph.D. may all contribute to this trend. Figure D-5 shows how graduates are dis-

[7] Finn, Michael G. "Stay Rates of Foreign Doctorate Recipients from U.S. Universities, 1995." Oak Ridge, Tenn.: Oak Ridge Institute for Science and Education, 1997.

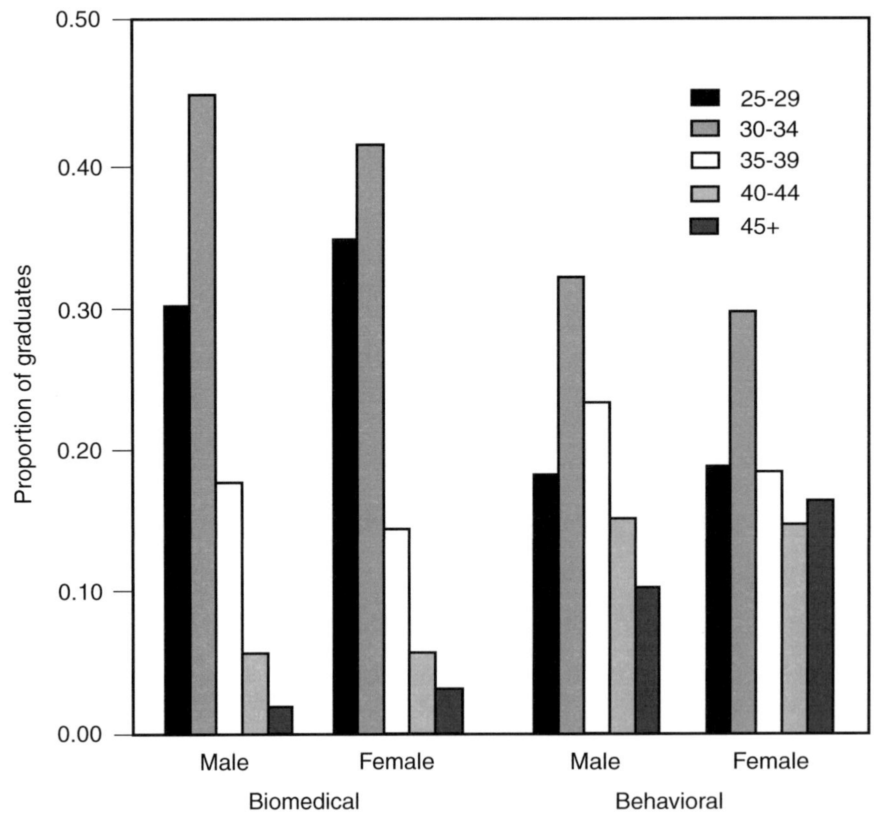

FIGURE D-5 Proportion of Ph.D. graduates in each age group by field and gender: 1990-96 averages. SOURCE: Data are from the Survey of Earned Doctorates.

tributed by age, using averages for the period 1990-96. The proportion of older graduates in behavioral research has reached quite a high level. Among female behavioral scientists particularly, graduates age 40 years and over make up almost a third of the total. These five-year age distributions will be used in the projections, converted to smoothed single-year distributions.

How soon these new graduates become employed is not known. Throughout the projections they are assumed to distribute across possible employment status immediately and in the same proportion as other graduates of their age already in the workforce or employed outside science in the year of their graduation.[8]

Entry Through Immigration

Ph.D.s who obtain their degrees abroad and then immigrate into the U.S. are not included in these data. Unlike foreign students who obtain Ph.D.s in the U.S., immigrants with Ph.D.s obtained abroad are not in such compendia as the Doctorate Records File. Their estimated numbers are reported in Table D-2 from the 1995 Survey of College Graduates, which followed up those identified in the 1990 census. Immigrant Ph.D.s do make a contribution to the workforce, particularly in biomedical research, where they make up about a tenth of the number of U.S. Ph.D.s. Their numbers, broken down by age and employment status, will therefore be added to the base population.

These data on the stock of Ph.D. immigrants cannot be used to determine their flow, because this survey does not have dates of entry into the U.S. Instead the 1993 Survey of College Graduates will be used. Both surveys relied on the 1990 census as a frame and covered the same universe. The 1993 survey, which is closer to the date of entry for the immigrants, is therefore preferable.

The immigrants in 1993 were broken down by age, field, and gender, as well as date of entry into the U.S., and are coded in the survey file as before 1981, 1981-82, 1983-84, 1985-86, or 1987-90. The size of each cohort when it entered the country (at the midpoint of period of entry) was estimated using assumed mortality and retirement rates described below. (See the Technical Note later in this appendix for an explanation of the process of reverse survival. The cohort entering before 1981 was excluded because of the indefinite dates of entry.) Inferring the original number of entrants this way has little effect on the number of younger immigrant Ph.D.s but can substantially increase the number of older ones beyond the numbers reported in cross-sectional surveys.

Given the small number of immigrants in the survey, estimated annual numbers by period are irregular, including implausible zero totals for some groups in some periods. A strong upward trend in total immigrants across all ages does appear over time in biomedical research, and an upward trend may also be possible in behavioral research (see Figure D-6). Depending on how growth is estimated and for which groups, the annual growth rate for immigrant Ph.D.s over the period 1981-90 is around 10 percent to14 percent, a trend that might be compared to the recently

[8] In these calculations the 1995 graduates are assumed to enter the workforce and be counted in the figures for 1995 described previously. Graduates in 1996, for whom data are also available, are added to the workforce in 1996, and the scenarios based on regressions described above are used to give total graduates in subsequent years.

TABLE D-2 Immigrant Ph.D.s by Employment Status, Field, and Gender, 1995

	Biomedical Ph.D.s		Behavioral Ph.D.s	
Employment Status	Males	Females	Males	Females
Employed	5,471	2,147	355	407
Unemployed	135	176	0	0
Not in labor force	120	406	0	89
Total potential workforce	5,726	2,729	355	496
Outside science	1,413	605	1,330	380
Retired	471	71	0	60

SOURCE: Data are from the Survey of College Graduates.

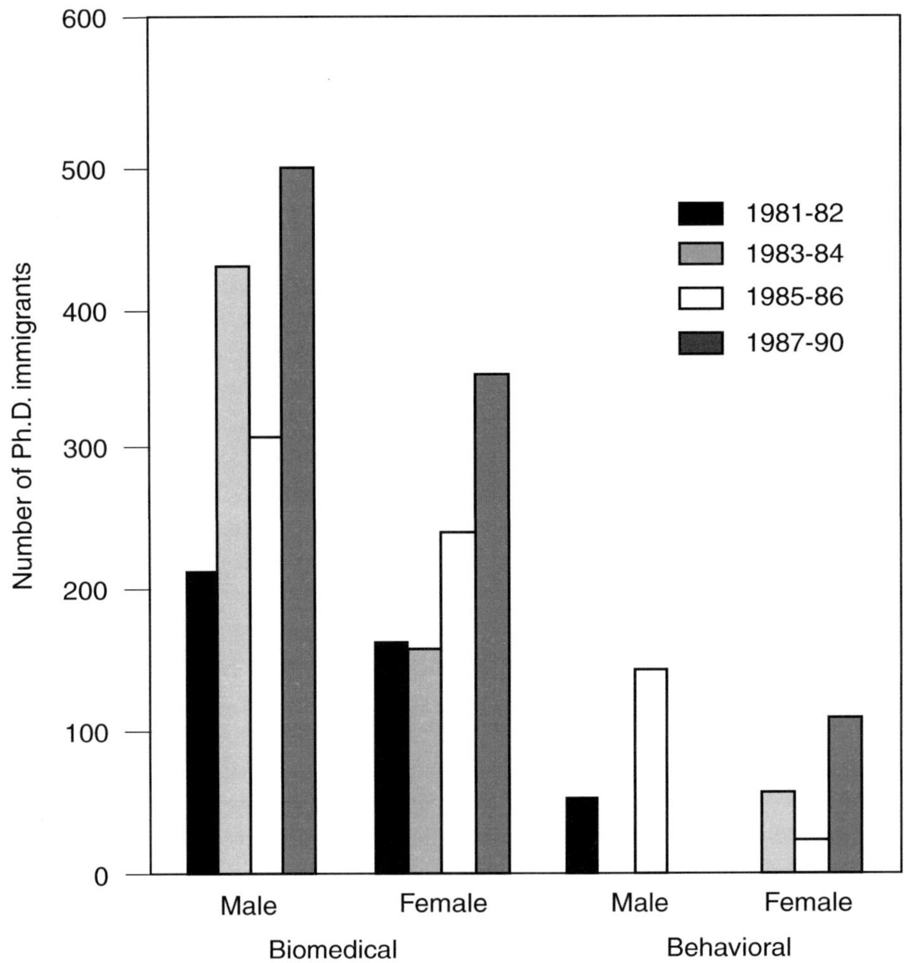

FIGURE D-6 Estimated annual Ph.D. immigrants by period, field, and gender. SOURCE: Data are from the Survey of College Graduates.

increased proportion of U.S. Ph.D.s awarded to foreign nationals.

Averaging across periods suggests that 600 biomedical scientists and 100 behavioral scientists immigrate annually. In biomedical research, about two-thirds of these are under 35 years of age when they immigrate, in contrast to behavioral research, where only a third are under 35.

To project immigrant flow, annual numbers by age were averaged across periods, again leaving out the period before 1981, and age patterns were smoothed using five-year moving averages. These numbers will be held constant and paired with the "medium-growth" projections of graduates in the central projections, which will therefore incorporate the typical migration levels for 1981-90. Alternatively, immigrants may be excluded altogether; this option will be paired with the "low-growth" projections of graduates. (For the first year at least, eliminating immigrants has about the same effect on total numbers as moving from medium to low graduate projections.) A third option is rising immigration. Immigrant Ph.D.s will be assumed to increase at an annual exponential growth rate of 0.10; this option will be paired with the "high-growth" projections of graduates. All these projections of future migration trends tend to understate the impact of immigration. The medium and high options are based on the average over a decade rather than on the high point reached closer to the start of the projection. More moderate growth is posited in the high option (rather than 14 percent) because of uncertainty about whether such growth would be sustainable. In the high option the annual number of immigrant biomedical scientists already rises from 600 to 1,600.

Other Entries, Exits, and Transitions

Other ways to enter or exit from the potential workforce must be examined to establish projection parameters. To complete the picture, change of status (for example, from employed to unemployed or not in the labor force) will also be examined.

The data to be considered, already used in determining the current workforce, are derived from the biennial Survey of Doctorate Recipients. Ph.D.s were classified by employment status in 1985 and their subsequent status in 1987 was determined. This tabulation was repeated for each succeeding two-year cycle. The data were then pooled across cycles to provide enough cases to support the estimation of age-specific transition rates.

Table D-3 collapses the data further across age groups to reveal the overall picture. For each group defined by major field and gender, the majority of Ph.D.s are employed at the beginning and end of each biennium. The next largest category includes those employed outside science, who make up 5 percent of such cases among biomedical Ph.D.s and 12 percent among behavioral Ph.D.s.

The most important transition results from mobility between employment in science and employment outside science. Almost 5 percent of those employed in science have shifted to jobs outside science two years later, whereas a third of those originally outside science have become employed in science. Those moving out of science, however, still outnumber those moving in, by a ratio of 5:3 overall. The peak ages for moving out of science are 39 to 49 years (see Figures D-7 and D-8).

Examined over time, job shifts into and out of science appear to rise and fall together in each field. The frequency of shifts is also correlated across fields and between males and females, which suggests the importance of market factors—perhaps the availability of university positions or research funds—affecting these fields. Over time the frequency of job shifts shows no apparent overall trend. Shifts appeared to reach a peak in 1991, which may have been due to economic conditions but could also have been the result of survey modifications.

The next most important transition is employment to retirement. In a typical two-year period, less than 3 percent of researchers make this transition (see Table D-3). The proportion retiring is of course strongly patterned by age; it is essentially zero below age 50 and rises quickly from age 60 on (see Figure D-9). Rates for females appear somewhat more volatile, possibly because of a smaller base, and may be slightly lower than for males, though the effect may be somewhat offset by the greater tendency for retired men to return to work. (Those who return to work are few overall and are essentially ignored here.) When examined for 5- and 10-year age groups among those 50 years old and over, retirement rates show no detectable trend over time.

Table D-3 indicates that transitions into and out of unemployment and into and out of not in the labor force involve relatively small numbers (though, like other reversible transitions, these might be understated given the two-year time frame). Moving into and out of the labor force is clearly more important among women in both fields, however. Substantially larger numbers of women than men leave the labor force. Under age 50, men outnumber women among the employed by 2-3 to 1. But women outnumber men by similar proportions among those who leave the labor force.

The data on Ph.D.s with U.S. degrees who reside abroad require clarification. Because of changes in survey methodology, changes in the status of these Ph.D.s are not available after 1991. Some Ph.D.s do seem to rejoin the U.S. workforce, but in the absence of data on current numbers abroad, one cannot reliably include this transition in the calculations.

Transition rates from these data were calculated for two-year age groups over two-year periods. Rates were estimated conditionally. For example, the rate for moving from employed to not in the labor force was estimated conditional on nonretirement (i.e., excluding those who retired). To facilitate projections, rates were converted to annual rates (using the square root of the survival rate) and smoothed using five-year moving averages. Smoothing was not applied to retirement rates; the peaks at ages 65 and 70, which already appear less sharp because of the biennial data, could reflect actual behavior.

Exit Through Death

Mortality rates cannot be estimated reliably from these surveys. Instead, life tables were used for TIAA/CREF "participants," mainly university employees and employees of nonprofit organizations. These tables indicate a life expectancy at birth of 74.1 years for males and 79.4 for females. For males the figure is slightly higher than estimates for the general population: 72.5,

TABLE D-3 Initial Employment Status and Status Two Years Later, Pooled 1985-95 Data (percent)

Final Employment Status	Initial Employment Status						
	Employed	Unemployed	Not in Labor Force	Outside Science	Retired	Abroad[a]	Total
			Male biomedical Ph.D.s				
Employed	80.7	0.4	0.2	1.6	0.3	0.3	83.4
Unemployed	0.5	0.1	0.0	0.1	0.0	0.0	0.8
Not in labor force	0.3	0.2	0.4	0.1	0.1	0.0	1.0
Outside science	2.7	0.1	0.0	2.1	0.1	0.0	5.1
Retired	1.8	1.2	0.1	0.1	4.7	0.0	7.8
Abroad	0.2	0.0	0.0	0.0	0.0	1.6	1.8
Total	86.3	2.1	0.7	4.0	5.1	1.9	100.0
Weighted cases[b]	(215,176)	(5,238)	(1,762)	(9,865)	(12,776)	(4,657)	(249,474)
			Female biomedical Ph.D.s				
Employed	74.6	0.9	0.9	2.1	0.1	0.3	78.9
Unemployed	1.0	0.2	0.2	0.1	0.0	0.0	1.6
Not in labor force	1.7	0.3	2.2	0.1	0.2	0.0	4.6
Outside science	3.7	0.3	0.2	3.5	0.0	0.0	7.7
Retired	0.8	0.9	0.1	0.2	3.9	0.0	5.9
Abroad	0.2	0.0	0.0	0.0	0.0	1.1	1.3
Total	82.0	2.7	3.8	6.0	4.2	1.4	100.0
Weighted cases[b]	(58,676)	(1,901)	(2,701)	(4,277)	(2,972)	(1,017)	(71,544)
			Male behavioral Ph.D.s				
Employed	71.4	0.2	0.2	3.2	0.4	0.2	75.6
Unemployed	0.4	0.3	0.1	0.1	0.0	0.0	0.9
Not in labor force	0.2	0.0	0.1	0.0	0.1	0.0	0.5
Outside science	4.9	0.1	0.1	6.7	0.2	0.0	11.9
Retired	2.4	0.0	0.1	0.4	4.2	0.0	7.1
Abroad	0.3	0.0	0.0	0.0	0.8	2.8	4.0
Total	79.6	0.6	0.7	10.5	5.6	3.0	100.0
Weighted cases[b]	(101,843)	(771)	(856)	(13,436)	(7,182)	(3,871)	(127,959)
			Female behavioral Ph.D.s				
Employed	69.8	1.0	0.7	3.0	0.1	0.3	74.9
Unemployed	1.1	0.5	0.2	0.1	0.0	0.1	2.0
Not in labor force	1.1	0.2	1.3	0.4	0.1	0.0	3.0
Outside science	5.8	0.3	0.4	7.7	0.0	0.0	14.3
Retired	1.0	0.0	0.2	0.1	2.5	0.0	3.9
Abroad	0.3	0.0	0.0	0.0	0.0	1.6	2.0
Total	79.1	2.0	2.8	11.4	2.7	2.0	100.0
Weighted cases[b]	(44,007)	(1,126)	(1,540)	(6,348)	(1,518)	(1,129)	(55,668)

[a] Data on those abroad were not collected in 1993 and 1995. This category therefore reflects 1985-91 data only and is almost certainly underestimated.

[b] As explained in the text, the number of cases is weighted to reflect the total population—for this table the combined population for five periods.

SOURCE: Data are estimated from the Survey of Doctorate Recipients.

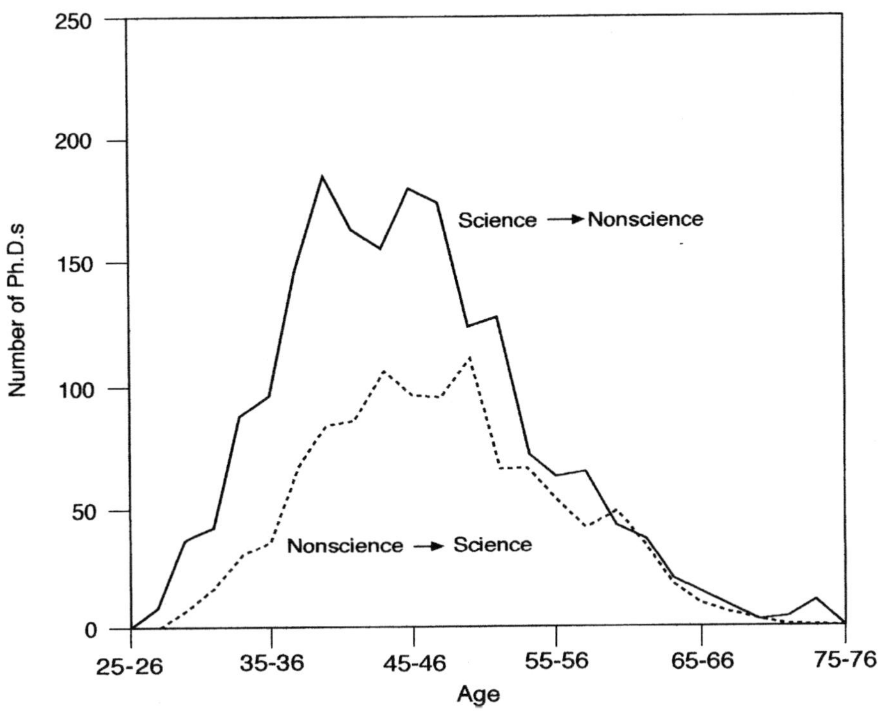

FIGURE D-7 Biennial shifts between science and nonscience jobs by age group: biomedical scientists, 1985-95 averages. SOURCE: Data are from the Survey of Doctorate Recipients.

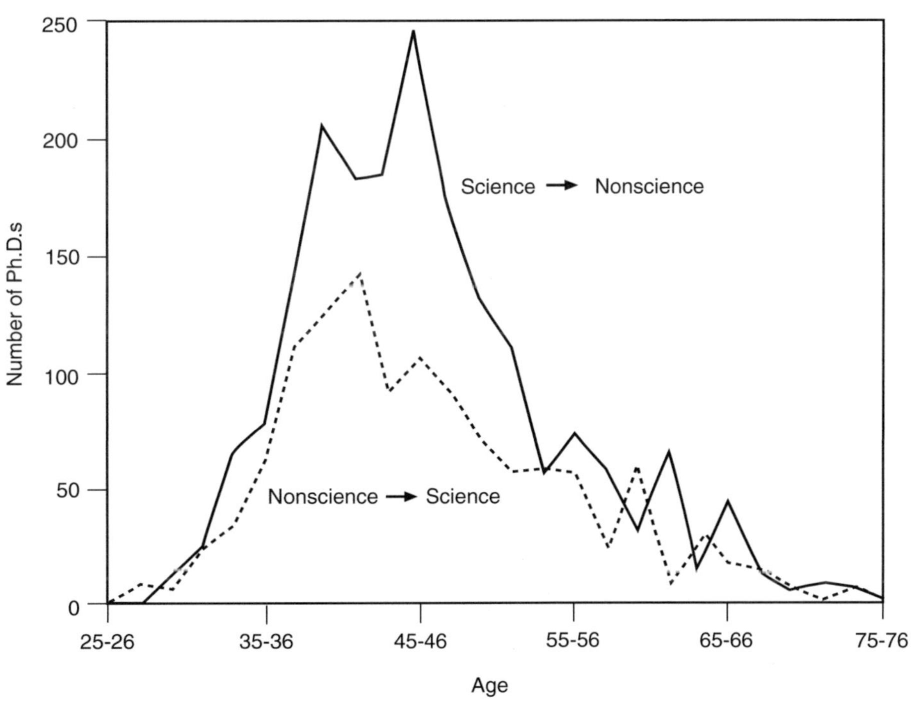

FIGURE D-8 Biennial shifts between science and nonscience jobs by age group: behavioral scientists, 1985-95 averages. SOURCE: Data are from the Survey of Doctorate Recipients.

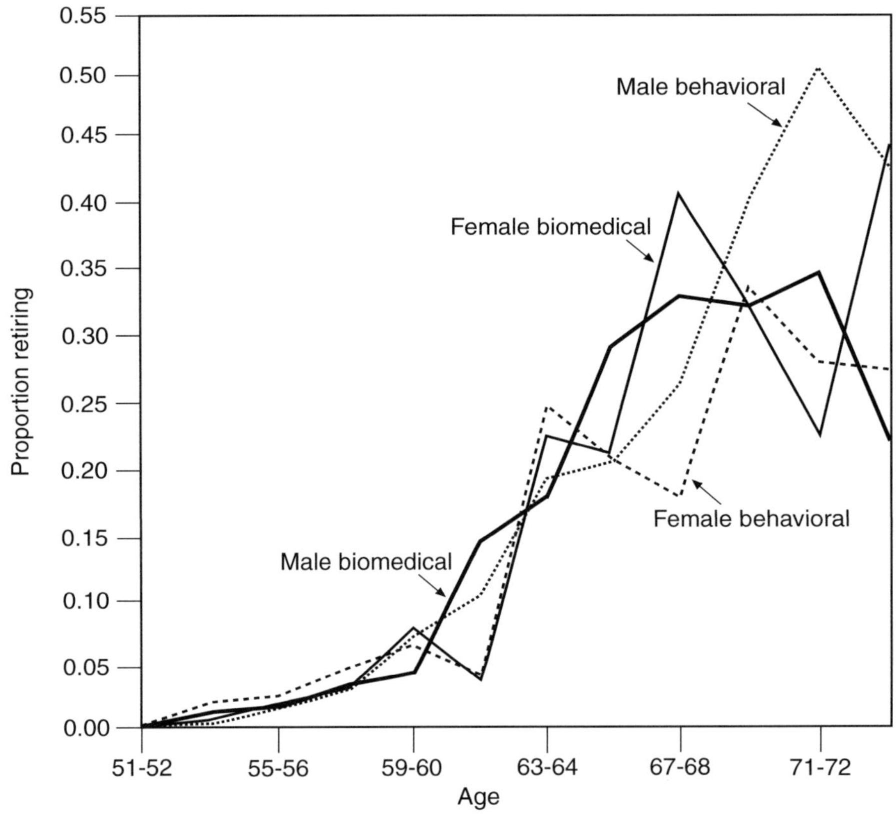

FIGURE D-9 Proportion retiring in two years among those employed in science by age, field, and gender: 1985-95 averages. SOURCE: Data are from the Survey of Doctorate Recipients.

according to the U.S. Census Bureau,[9] and 73.4, according to the U.N. Population Division.[10] One might well expect some such advantage in a more educated group. For females, however, the life expectancy estimate essentially matches estimates for the general population (79.3 and 80.1, according to the same two sources). Since data are not available by field or employment status, the same mortality rates are used for all groups.

PROJECTION RESULTS

Projection of the Workforce

Using the assumptions just outlined, 10-year workforce projections were constructed for each of four groups defined by field and gender. An initial overview of the results follows; details of the procedure are provided in the Technical Note later in this appendix.

Figure D-10 shows the workforce in biomedical and behavioral research over time. Data from 1985 to 1995 are derived from surveys, and data from 1995 on are projection results. Three alternative projections are shown, assuming high, medium, and low numbers of Ph.D. graduates (and corresponding high, medium, and low numbers of immigrant Ph.D.s as described above). The high and low projections are meant to set possible bounds on future trends rather than to reflect likely alternatives.

The workforce in biomedical research, which is 70 percent larger than that in behavioral research, is projected to grow more than three times as fast. The annual growth rate of the biomedical workforce over the period 1995-2005 is estimated at 3.4 percent in the medium projection and in the high and low projections at 4.4 and 2.2 percent. The workforce in behavioral research, on the other hand, will also grow (at 1.2 percent in the medium projection). In the high projection, an-

[9] U.S. Bureau of the Census. *Population Projections of the U.S. by Sex, Race, and Hispanic Origin: 1995 to 2050*. Washington, D.C.: U.S. Bureau of the Census, 1996.

[10] United Nations. *World Population Prospects 1950-2050: The 1998 Revision*. New York: UN, 1999.

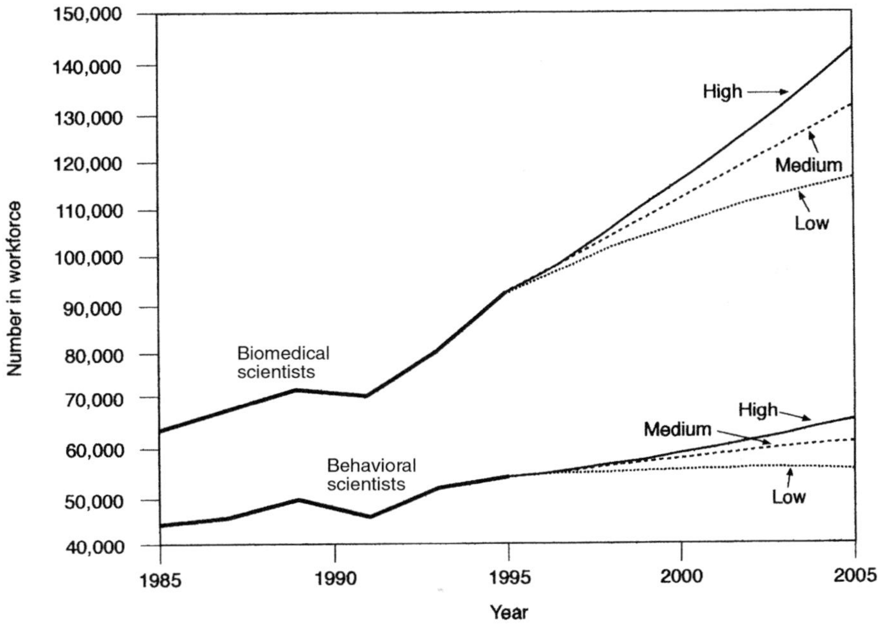

FIGURE D-10 Workforce projections with varying numbers of graduates: biomedical and behavioral scientists, 1985-2005. SOURCE: Data are from projections described in the text.

nual growth rises to 2.0 percent, but in the low projection annual growth over the entire period is barely positive at 0.3 percent, which reflects an initial slight increase to the year 2003 and a subsequent modest decline.

The medium annual growth rate in biomedical research is higher than that projected by the U.S. Bureau of Labor Statistics[11] for 1996-2006, which is 2.1 percent in the life sciences. For behavioral research, on the other hand, the medium rate is close to that estimated by the bureau, which is 0.9 percent in the social sciences. (The contrasts will be discussed further in the concluding section below.)

The projected growth for both fields may be understood as an extension of growth in the previous decade. In 1985-95 the biomedical research workforce (excluding immigrant Ph.D.s) grew 3.0 percent annually and the behavioral research workforce grew 1.2 percent annually. Projections, however, do not reproduce the variability in past trends. The apparent fluctuations in growth between 1985 and 1995—large increases at some points and occasional declines at others might be due to the complex weighting procedures, which vary among the surveys or to survey errors or sample variability. These data probably deserve closer examination, but projections nevertheless address the most important trends, around which considerable annual variation is possible.

Two qualifications are useful regarding Figure D-10 and subsequent figures. First, the 1995 estimates shown are smoothed and adjusted and so differ slightly from the biennial survey reports. Second, immigrants with Ph.D.s are included from 1995 on but not in the earlier survey data, which accounts for some increase.

The actual numbers from the medium projection, which assumes a medium trend in graduates and constant immigration, show differential growth between males and females (see Table D-4). Male biomedical scientists will increase by 17,200 and female biomedical scientists by 19,900 over the decade. In spite of its smaller base, the female workforce has an annual growth rate two and a half times as high as the male (5.7 percent versus 2.3 percent). In behavioral research the contrast is even sharper, since males are projected to decrease (by 1,300 over the decade) and females to increase (by 8,000).

Figures D-11 and D-12 show the composition of the workforce in each field in the medium projection, with males and females disaggregated among the employed, though not among the much smaller numbers of persons unemployed, not in the labor force, and outside science. The graphs illustrate the consistency with ear-

[11] U.S. Bureau of Labor Statistics, Office of Employment Projections. "National Industry-Occupation Employment Projections 1996-2006." Washington, D.C.: U.S. Department of Labor, 1997.

TABLE D-4 Projected Ph.D. Workforce and Ph.D.s Outside Science, Assuming Medium Trend in Graduates and Constant Immigration, 1995-2005

	Biomedical Scientists				Behavioral Scientists			
	Male		Female		Male		Female	
Year	Workforce	Outside Science	Workforce	Outside Science	Workforce	Outside Science	Workforce	Outside Science
1995	65,615	6,500	25,825	3,350	31,315	6,477	21,862	3,900
1996	67,668	5,931	27,775	3,360	31,204	6,285	22,628	4,189
1997	69,620	5,544	29,657	3,401	31,153	6,134	23,404	4,458
1998	71,480	5,308	31,570	3,487	31,107	5,996	24,199	4,702
1999	73,260	5,188	33,510	3,607	31,037	5,865	25,008	4,925
2000	74,959	5,154	35,470	3,751	30,931	5,742	25,824	5,125
2001	76,604	5,176	37,455	3,912	30,809	5,628	26,633	5,304
2002	78,211	5,232	39,480	4,084	30,678	5,520	27,447	5,467
2003	79,781	5,315	41,532	4,269	30,517	5,419	28,263	5,628
2004	81,309	5,415	43,609	4,465	30,298	5,306	29,062	5,788
2005	82,792	5,525	45,719	4,674	30,043	5,192	29,838	5,943

SOURCE: Data are from projections described in the text.

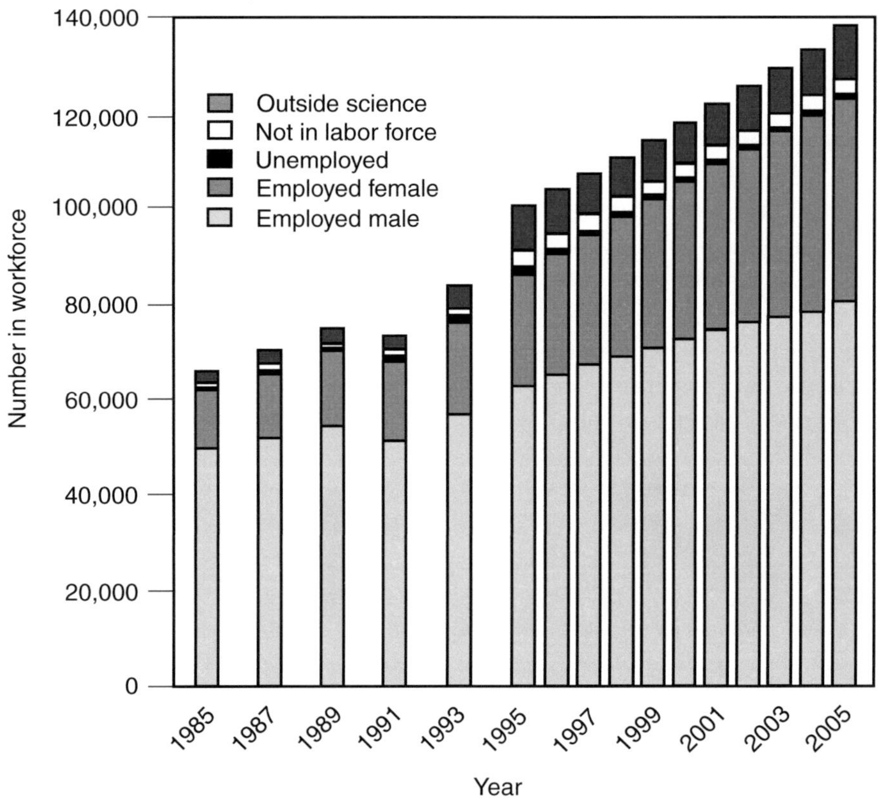

FIGURE D-11 Reported and projected workforce by employment status and Ph.D.s outside science: biomedical scientists, 1985-2005. SOURCE: Data are from the Survey of Doctorate Recipients and projections described in the text.

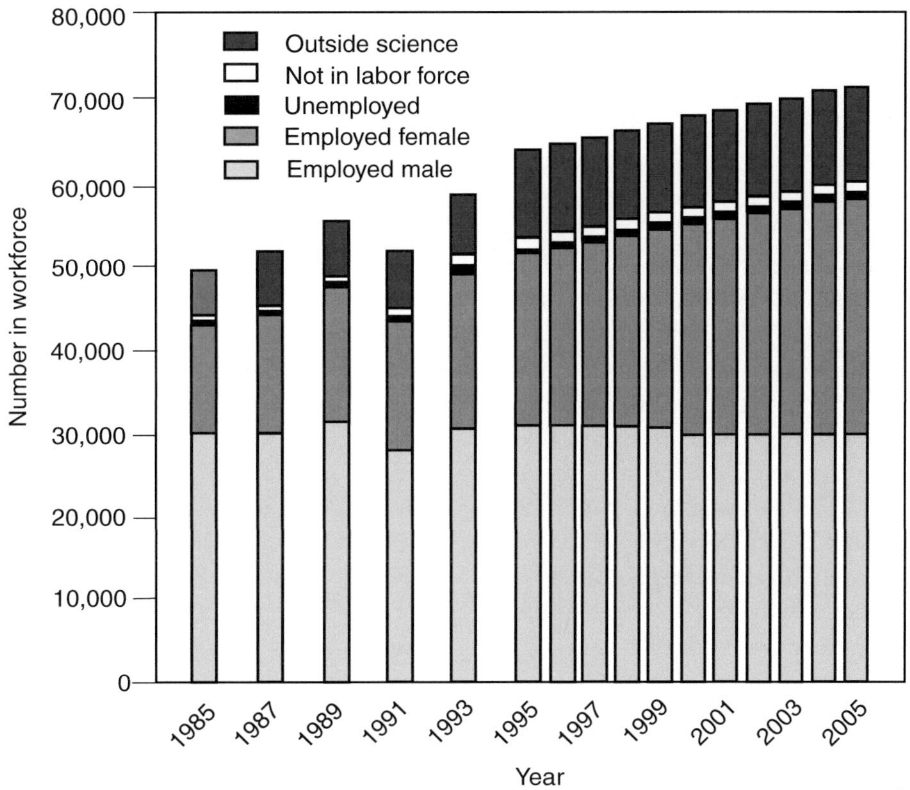

FIGURE D-12 Reported and projected workforce by employment status and Ph.D.s outside science: behavioral scientists, 1985-2005. SOURCE: Data are from the Survey of Doctorate Recipients and projections described in the text.

lier trends of projected trends in the workforce. They also underline the contrast between biomedical research, where each component of the workforce is growing vigorously, and behavioral research, where employed males—the largest component—are declining in numbers.

Of the smaller components of the potential workforce, the unemployed are so few in number as to be barely visible in these figures. At 1.7 percent of the potential biomedical research workforce in 1995, their proportion was elevated over earlier levels, and the level after 10 years is projected to settle around 0.7 percent. Among behavioral researchers, on the other hand, the 1995 unemployment level of 0.8 percent is sharply lower than in previous years, and the level at which it settles after a decade is 1.4 percent.

Those not in the labor force, on the other hand, are at least twice as numerous as the unemployed. Their numbers rose sharply in the mid-1990s and are projected to stabilize. In 1995 those not in the labor force composed 3.6 percent of the potential workforce among biomedical Ph.D.s. By 2005 they will make up 2.6 percent of the total, though they will still be more numerous than in 1995. Their projected decline as a proportion of the workforce will signal a return to pre-1993 levels; the simultaneous increase in numbers is possible mainly because of the changing gender composition of the workforce, since 8 percent of women but only 2 percent of men are not in the labor force. Among behavioral researchers, the percentage not in the labor force starts at 3.0 in 1995 but also reaches 2.6 by 2005. The contrast between men and women is similar.

The final group in Figures D-11 and D-12 shows those employed outside science, who are not considered part of the research workforce. As with those not in the labor force, their numbers increased sharply in the mid-1990s. They are projected to continue to increase, though only slowly. From the equivalent of 11 percent of the biomedical research workforce in 1995 they will fall to 8 percent by 2005. In behavioral research those outside science were equivalent to 20 percent of the workforce in 1995 and will be 19 percent of the workforce by 2005.

The median age of the biomedical research workforce, at 45.5 years in 1995, has risen three years since 1985. Over the projection period it will rise less than a year, to 46.2 years by 2005. The rise will be relatively small because more women, who tend to be younger, will be entering the workforce than men. Women will increase from 28 percent to 36 percent of the workforce (see Figure D-13). Their median age was 4 years less than that of men in 1995 and will be 5 years less by 2005.

The behavioral research workforce has been aging more rapidly. The median age rose 5.5 years from 1985, to stand at 48.8 years by 1995. Before the year 2000 it will cross the 50-year mark and by 2005 will stand at 52.4 years. Figure D-14 shows somewhat contrasting patterns for males and females. Males aged 40-59 will be the only broad age group to actually decline in size over the projection, whereas males 60 years old and older will increase 70 percent in a decade. Among females, aging will be reflected mainly in shifts within the broad age group 40 to 59. Females were 41 percent of the potential workforce in 1995 and by 2005 will be half of the total.

These changes in workforce composition result from entries and exits represented in Figure D-15, which show movements not in absolute numbers but as a proportion of the potential workforce by sex. Exits are represented with negative signs. Because the picture does not change greatly across the years of the projection, the year 2000 is used for illustration.

The entrance of graduates is projected to be clearly the most important movement; those actually entering the workforce in 2000 will represent the equivalent of 4 percent of the workforce in each field. Job shifts into and out of science will also be important, with shifts in each direction equivalent to 2 percent of the workforce in biomedical research and 3 percent of the workforce in behavioral research. However, inward and outward job shifts are projected to be almost equal in most cases and to cancel each other out—a change from the excess outward movement in the late 1980s and early 1990s. Annual retirements will account for 1 percent of the

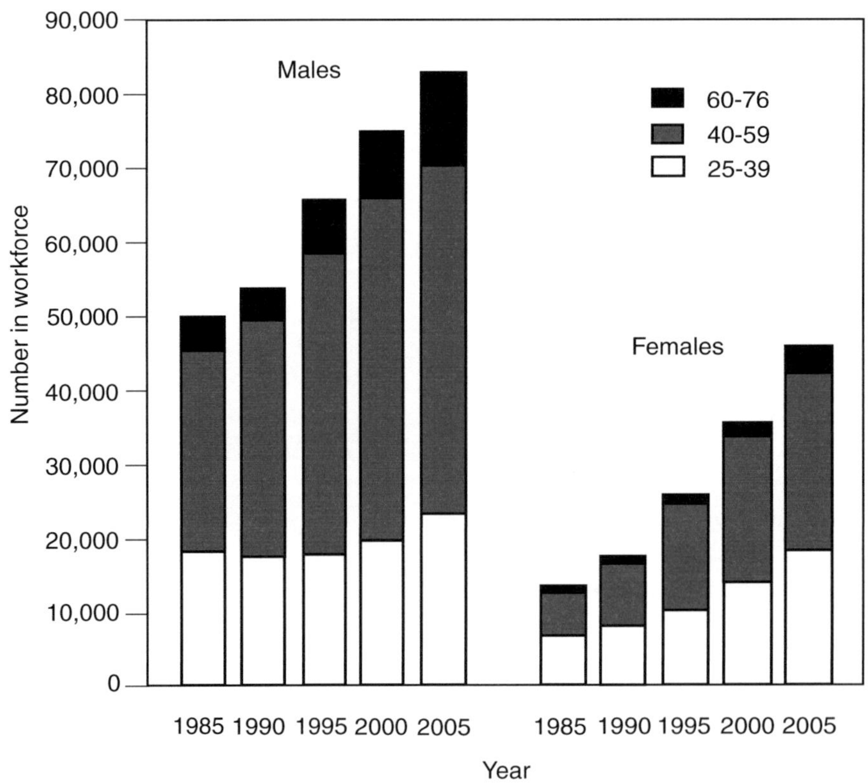

FIGURE D-13 Reported and projected age distribution of workforce: biomedical scientists, 1985-2005. SOURCE: Data are from the Survey of Doctorate Recipients and projections described in the text.

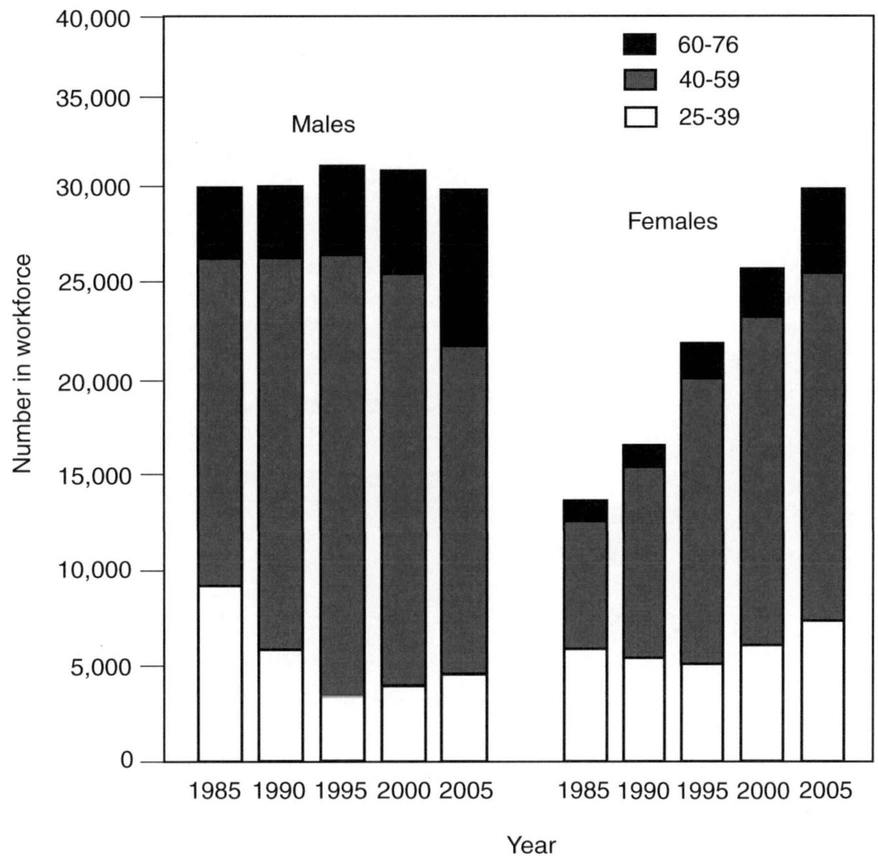

FIGURE D-14 Reported and projected age distribution of workforce: behavioral scientists, 1985-2005. SOURCE: Data are from the Survey of Doctorate Recipients and projections described in the text.

biomedical research workforce and 2 percent of the behavioral research workforce; in each field, annual deaths will be about a quarter of this figure. With graduates projected at more than three times the number of retirements in biomedical research and almost twice the number of retirements in behavioral research, the reasons for expecting continued workforce growth are clear.

The importance of some of these changes varies by gender. New graduates as a proportion of the workforce by sex and field are more likely to be female than male; the proportion of men who retire is twice that of women; and the proportion of deaths is three times greater among men than among women. The ratio of entering graduates to exiting retirees, therefore, varies from more than 8:1 among female biomedical scientists to 1:1 among male behavioral scientists.

If, however, the greater numbers of graduates and rising immigration assumed in the high projection were to occur, the result would be significantly more growth (see Table D-5 and Figure D-10). The potential workforce grows 55 percent in biomedical research in a decade, according to this projection, and 22 percent in behavioral research. The alternative low projection (see Table D-6) shows these workforces growing 25 percent and 3 percent, respectively, over the decade. As a proportion of the workforce, graduates in the high projection are half a percentage point more numerous than in the medium projection (in both fields), and graduates in the low projection are half a percentage point less numerous. Immigrants vary slightly less. Other entries and exits do not vary from their proportions in the medium projection.

Graduates Needed for a Constant Workforce

Instead of asking how the potential workforce will grow, one might ask what hypothetical number of Ph.D. graduates would be needed to keep the workforce constant. This question can be answered by simulating

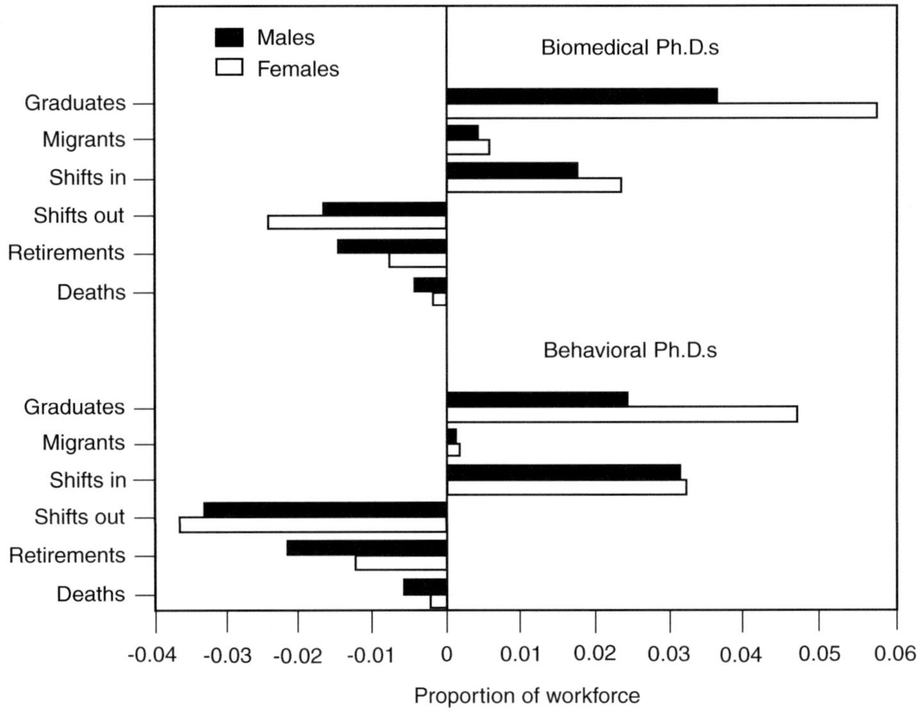

FIGURE D-15 Entries and exits as a proportion of the workforce by field and gender, 2000. SOURCE: Data are from projections described in the text.

workforces staying at their 1995 size for each of the four groups (by field and gender) for a decade (as described in the Technical Note later in this appendix). In these simulations the number of 1996 graduates will be allowed to vary from reported numbers, unlike in the previous projections. The age distribution of graduates will again be held constant and immigration will also be assumed to be constant. Other assumptions, espe-

TABLE D-5 Projected Ph.D. Workforce and Ph.D.s Outside Science, Assuming High Trend in Graduates and Rising Immigration, 1995-2005

	Biomedical Ph.D.s				Behavioral Ph.D.s			
	Male		Female		Male		Female	
Year	Workforce	Outside Science	Workforce	Outside Science	Workforce	Outside Science	Workforce	Outside Science
1995	65,615	6,500	25,825	3,350	31,315	6,477	21,862	3,900
1996	67,704	5,933	27,798	3,362	31,214	6,285	22,638	4,190
1997	69,913	5,556	29,961	3,423	31,275	6,143	23,502	4,466
1998	72,123	5,337	32,252	3,534	31,379	6,016	24,415	4,723
1999	74,350	5,241	34,674	3,685	31,502	5,900	25,382	4,962
2000	76,599	5,240	37,228	3,866	31,635	5,797	26,398	5,184
2001	78,910	5,304	39,924	4,071	31,798	5,710	27,452	5,392
2002	81,300	5,413	42,783	4,300	32,001	5,635	28,559	5,595
2003	83,780	5,558	45,790	4,554	32,227	5,572	29,711	5,803
2004	86,356	5,732	48,957	4,835	32,453	5,504	30,898	6,022
2005	89,032	5,926	52,296	5,144	32,703	5,441	32,113	6,248

SOURCE: Data are from projections described in the text.

TABLE D-6 Projected Ph.D. Workforce and Ph.D.s Outside Science, Assuming Low Trend in Graduates and No Immigration, 1995-2005

	Biomedical Ph.D.s				Behavioral Ph.D.s			
	Male		Female		Male		Female	
Year	Workforce	Outside Science	Workforce	Outside Science	Workforce	Outside Science	Workforce	Outside Science
1995	65,615	6,500	25,825	3,350	31,315	6,477	21,862	3,900
1996	67,318	5,915	27,541	3,346	31,128	6,279	22,534	4,187
1997	68,741	5,505	28,960	3,358	30,909	6,115	23,143	4,444
1998	70,025	5,243	30,340	3,413	30,664	5,962	23,746	4,679
1999	71,176	5,093	31,679	3,498	30,371	5,813	24,339	4,890
2000	72,190	5,027	32,964	3,604	30,011	5,668	24,913	5,076
2001	73,097	5,014	34,206	3,719	29,604	5,529	25,458	5,234
2002	73,907	5,035	35,412	3,841	29,148	5,392	25,984	5,366
2003	74,622	5,078	36,566	3,965	28,624	5,257	26,479	5,482
2004	75,235	5,136	37,667	4,090	28,000	5,104	26,935	5,582
2005	75,743	5,198	38,724	4,216	27,303	4,944	27,338	5,664

SOURCE: Data are from projections described in the text.

cially regarding transition rates, will be the same as in the preceding projections.

Under these conditions, the numbers of graduates that would keep workforce sizes constant would be smaller than the current numbers. This is illustrated in Table D-7, which shows required numbers (without subtracting those who would leave the U.S. after graduation). The negative numbers that appear in one col-

TABLE D-7 Graduates Needed to Produce a Constant Workforce or a Workforce with Fixed Growth, by Field and Gender, 1996-2005

	Biomedical Ph.D.s				Behavioral Ph.D.s			
	Male		Female		Male		Female	
Year	Constant Workforce	Fixed Growth	Constant Workforce	Fixed Growth	Constant Workforce	Fixed Growth	Constant Workforce	Constant Growth
1995[a]	2,955		2,125		1,013		1,388	
1996	684	1,285	−38	201	1,077	1,388	511	716
1997	761	1,373	−43	198	994	1,296	480	691
1998	902	1,525	−5	239	982	1,290	462	678
1999	1,040	1,673	39	285	1,002	1,315	449	667
2000	1,185	1,828	97	346	1,041	1,361	450	671
2001	1,301	1,952	146	397	1,062	1,388	468	692
2002	1,406	2,065	186	439	1,083	1,414	472	701
2003	1,511	2,178	240	496	1,127	1,462	486	719
2004	1,623	2,299	295	556	1,209	1,550	512	748
2005	1,745	2,429	338	602	1,263	1,612	544	787

NOTE: The fixed-growth simulation uses growth rates for the U.S. labor force as a whole: 0.8 percent annually for males, 1.3 percent for females.

[a]Actual, for comparison.

SOURCE: Data are from projections described in the text.

umn suggest that in those years, even with no graduates, the workforce would still expand. (The fixed-growth option shown in the table will be explained below.)

These projections show that if the workforce is not to expand, the number of graduates in biomedical research, in particular, must fall precipitously from 5,100 in 1995 to 650 in 1996. Even by 2005 the required graduates for a constant workforce would still be fewer than half the number of 1995 graduates. In behavioral research the decline in graduates, if a constant workforce were maintained, would be less extreme but still marked. Graduates would have to fall from 2,400 in 1995 to 1,600 in 1996 and increase only slightly by 2005. Table D-7 shows the required number of male graduates rising slightly above their 1995 level, but this increase would be more than offset by the decrease in female graduates.

The numbers of graduates that would produce a constant workforce are well below those assumed in the previous projections (see Figures D-16 and D-17). Even the low projection predicts a larger number of graduates, except for behavioral scientists at the very end of the projection period. To keep the workforce constant, therefore, would require a sharp discontinuity with previous trends, which are based on earlier surveys and shown in the figures.

In these constant-workforce simulations, each of the four groups is projected separately. The ratio of males to females in the workforce, therefore, is constrained not to change. The workforce in a field could of course still be held constant if women replaced departing men, or vice versa. One might then speak simply of 1,600 spaces to fill in the behavioral research workforce in 2000, whether by men or women. The gender of the individuals who fill these spaces would not affect the size of the workforce in that year but could affect its size in later years, since men and women enter the workforce at different ages and have different transition rates.

If women replaced men, would more or fewer graduates be required to maintain a constant workforce? Any difference would appear to be minor at best because various factors tend to cancel each other out. Mainly because of later retirement and also because of lower mortality, female Ph.D.s spend on average more time in the scientific workforce: 29 years for females versus 28 years for males in biomedical research, for instance.

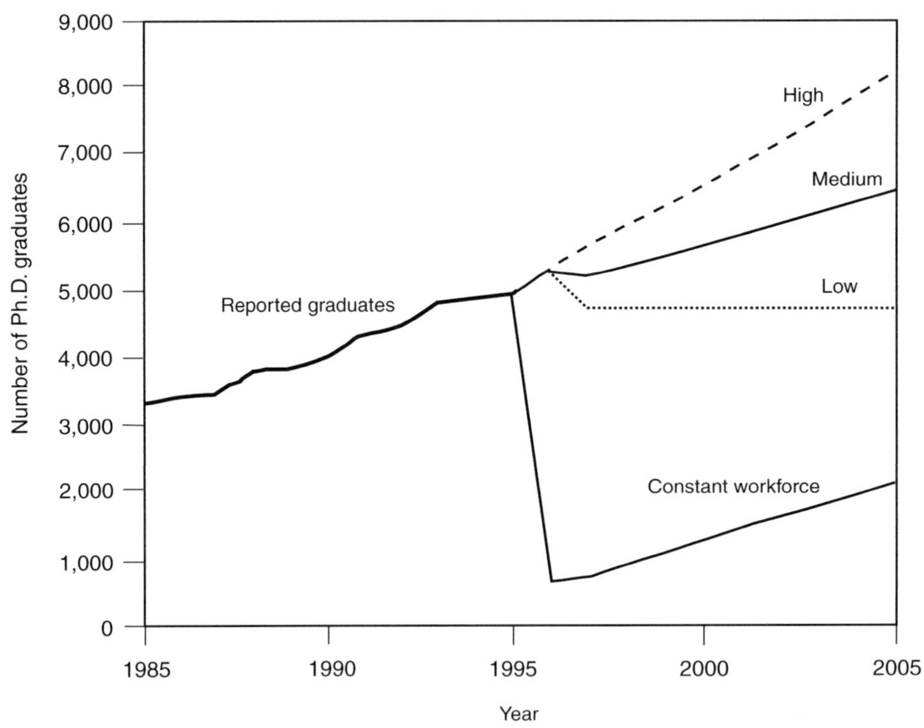

FIGURE D-16 Reported graduates and alternative projections: biomedical scientists, 1985-2005. SOURCE: Data are from the Survey of Earned Doctorates and projections described in the text.

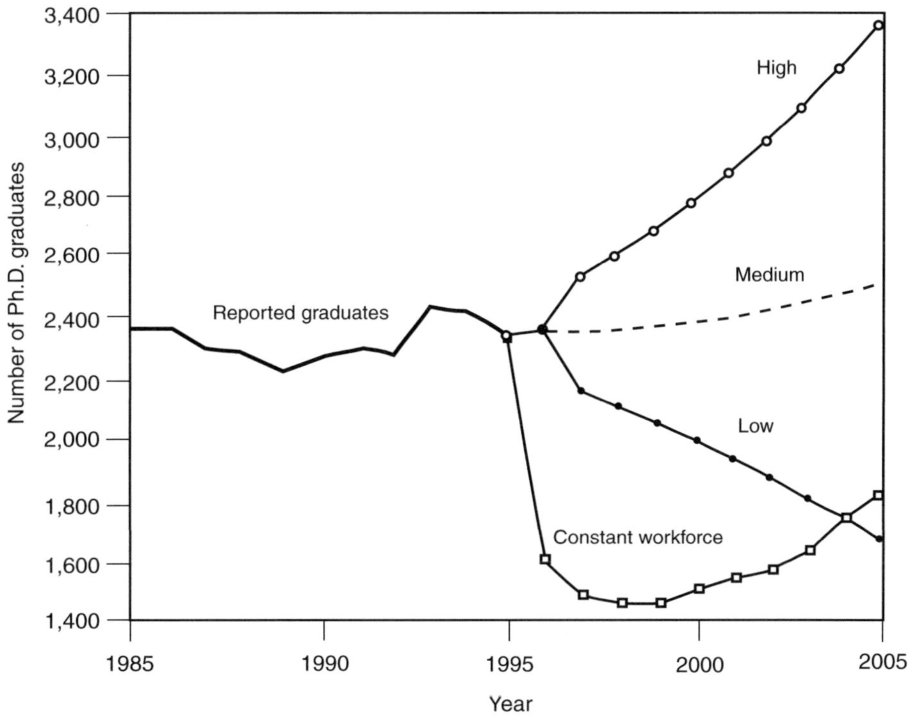

FIGURE D-17 Reported graduates and alternative projections: behavioral scientists, 1985-2005. SOURCE: Data are from the Survey of Earned Doctorates and projections described in the text.

(These estimates are based on the age distribution of graduates in 1995 and on constant transition rates as defined earlier and take into account possible emigration right after graduation.) If actual employment is considered, the advantage shifts to males (who are employed almost one year longer) in biomedical research. Furthermore, women work part-time more often (a factor not in the projections), which reduces the advantage even more. Overall, replacing men with women makes little difference in the projection period and, probably, even in the longer term.

The number of graduates required to maintain a constant workforce of biomedical scientists would rise if Ph.D. immigration were eliminated. Even under this unlikely assumption, however, the number would still be less than current graduation levels. Allowing immigration to rise, on the other hand, would require a further reduction in U.S. graduates. The effects of altering migration assumptions in either direction, however, are fairly small. Changing immigration assumptions for behavioral scientists makes even less difference because immigrants are fewer.

If the overall size of the workforce were to increase, the number of required graduates would naturally be higher than just estimated—how much higher would depend on the growth rates. Fixing the rates at 0.8 percent annual growth for men and 1.3 percent for women—the projected growth rates for the U.S. labor force as a whole[12]—would still imply reductions in graduates (see Table D-7).

For biomedical scientists, the required number of graduates would have to decline substantially—to 1,500 initially, fewer than a third of 1995 graduates. These numbers would double in a decade, but they would stay well below 1995 levels. For behavioral scientists, the required number of graduates would stay close to 1995 levels. A midperiod dip of up to 20 percent would be offset by a later recovery back to the 1995 level.

Graduate Projections and Enrollment

These projections of Ph.D. graduates have been made without reference to enrollments because, as

[12] Fullerton, Howard N. "The Labor Force in 2006: Slowing Down and Changing Composition." *Monthly Labor Review* 120, no. 11 (1997): 23-38.

noted earlier, enrollment in a given year does not predict the number that will eventually graduate. Enrollment ultimately does set limits on graduates, however, and looking at these limits may suggest whether and how enrollments may need to change.

As also noted earlier, the number of enrollees in a given year has been generally between 1.4 and 2.8 times the number of graduates six years later in these two fields for a decade. Whether the ratio for any given cohort will be closer to the high or the low end may not be predictable; however these figures may establish rough upper and lower limits on the number of future graduates.

These limits are illustrated for biomedical researchers in Figure D-18. The actual number of graduates year by year consistently remained within the limits but moved continuously toward the upper limit through the 1980s and early 1990s. The medium projection maintains this upward movement but keeps the number within the limits set by enrollment. (The upper limit of enrollment will be approached fairly closely toward the end of the projection.) Nevertheless, if graduate enrollments in biomedical research remain constant in 1998 and 1999, the medium projection should be achievable in 2004 and 2005 without breaching the upper limit.

The fixed-growth simulation, on the other hand, would drop the number of graduates below the lower limit set by enrollment. This means that if the biomedical research workforce grew only at the rate of the U.S. labor force, considerably smaller proportions of those enrolled in recent years would have to graduate than at any point in the preceding decade.

A similar representation of the behavioral research workforce considers fewer years, since it excludes earlier enrollment data that do not distinguish behavioral researchers from clinical psychologists (see Figure D-19). Both the medium projection of graduates and the fixed-growth projection provide figures that lie comfortably within the limits set by recent enrollments. Only a sharp one- or two-year decline in enrollment of at least 20 percent (unprecedented in recent years) would hamper the attainment of the projected number of graduates and even then only for the last two years of the projection.

In behavioral research, considerable leeway exists for the trend in graduates to change either upward or

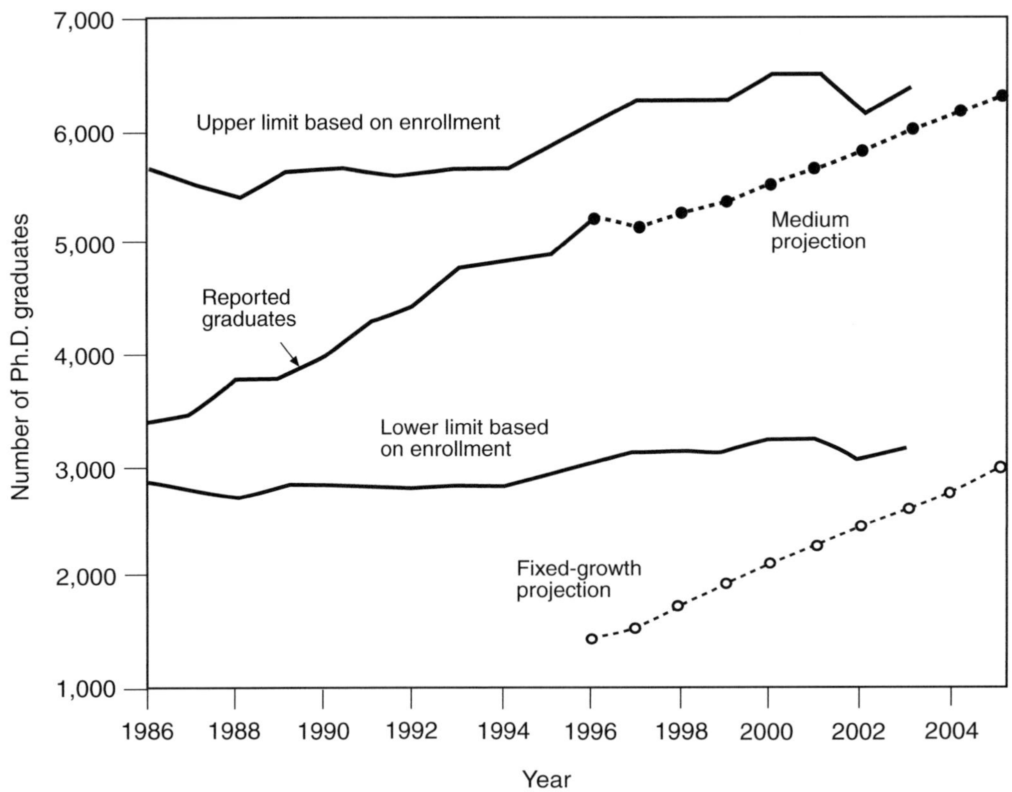

FIGURE D-18 Reported and projected graduates and limits set by enrollment lagged six years: biomedical scientists, 1986-2005. SOURCE: Data are from the Survey of Earned Doctorates and estimates and projections described in the text.

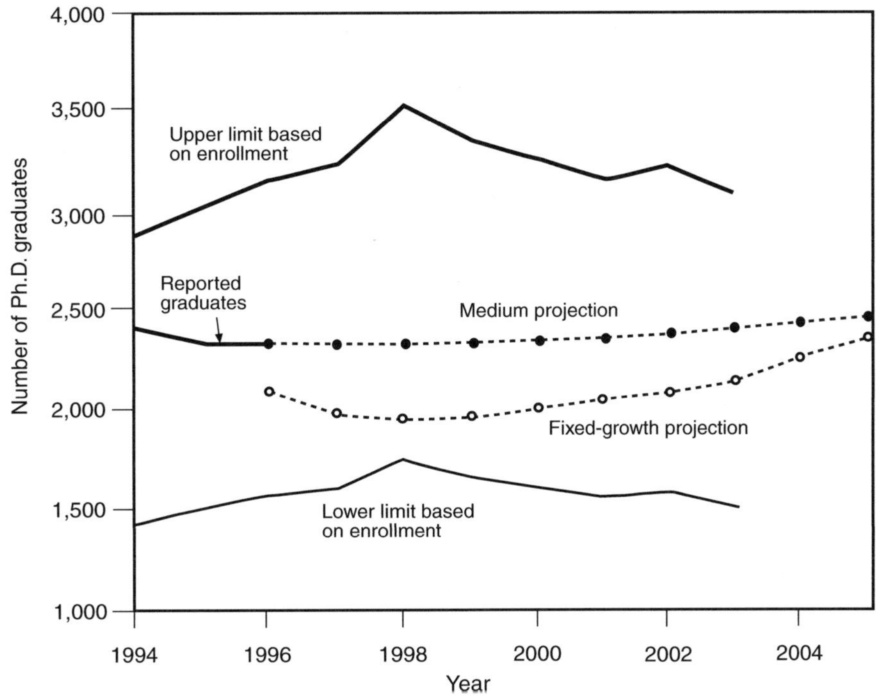

FIGURE D-19 Reported and projected graduates and limits set by enrollment lagged six years: behavioral scientists, 1994-2005. SOURCE: Data are from the Survey of Earned Doctorates and estimates and projections described in the text.

downward without altering enrollment. Even 3 percent annual growth, which is three times the projected rate (similar to the growth in the biomedical research workforce), could be accommodated by constant enrollments and would require only relatively moderate and historically achievable changes in the ratio of graduates to preceding enrollments.

IMPLICATIONS AND REFINEMENTS

If recent experience is a proper guide, the Ph.D. workforce in biomedical and behavioral research will continue to grow. In each field the current number of Ph.D. graduates substantially exceeds the number needed for a workforce of constant size. In addition, in biomedical research the number of graduates is clearly rising. Given current enrollment rates in graduate programs in the basic biomedical fields, the numbers of Ph.D. graduates are likely to at least continue at current levels for the next few years, or even increase. These conclusions are drawn from several projections. These are not meant as forecasts; the implications of a set of predefined assumptions have simply been worked out. Assumptions were chosen that reflect the recent behavior of the workforce, but no claim can be made that this behavior will in fact be replicated in the future. Dramatic changes in movement into and out of science or substantial variation in entering graduates or immigrants could presumably change the picture. The recent historical record suggests considerable biennial variation in the size of the workforce, variation not factored into the projections and deserving closer study.

Labor demand and education subsidy factors have not been incorporated into the model used here, though they could be important if substantial future discontinuities with recent experience occur. The employment outlook in these fields, the funding available for graduate education and research, and the status of immigrants and foreign students are all matters on which no judgment has been passed. In principle, such factors could be incorporated as predictors of entry and exit into the workforce, thus refining the projections.

Demand factors will constrain growth in these fields, if the workforce projections of the Bureau of Labor Statistics[13] are accurate. The bureau's projections are primarily driven by demand, proceeding from aggregate economic growth to commodity requirements to

[13] U.S. Bureau of Labor Statistics. *Handbook of Methods*. Washington, D.C.: U.S. Department of Labor, 1997.

the implied growth in specific industries. Projected industry trends are then converted into trends in occupations using a matrix relating over 250 industries to 500 occupational categories.[14] As noted above, for the categories corresponding most closely to those used here, bureau projections show growth rates only two-thirds as high as the medium projections here for biomedical scientists and three-fourths as high for behavioral scientists. The demand for researchers in these fields, therefore, is projected by the bureau to fall short of the supply projected here. If that turns out to be the case, the numbers of students entering these fields would presumably decline. Whether this decline would be timely and whether it would be too much or too little to avoid increased unemployment or underemployment is impossible to predict.

The transition rates and other input data and assumptions used here have substantial limitations and could in principle be improved in various ways. In particular, future forecasts of the research workforce would benefit from better information on employment outside science, immigration, foreign students, and the clinical research workforce. Historical trends in employment outside science cannot be thoroughly assessed due to data limitations, but some members of the Ph.D. workforce appear to move into and out of science jobs. The accuracy of the model could be improved through better information about such job shifts and the specific employment fields involved, as well as through further analysis of these trends. Data on immigrant Ph.D.s, who are roughly equivalent to a tenth of the workforce in biomedical research, should also be examined more closely. Their numbers and rates of increase have been estimated from quite limited data, and the factors that will affect their future numbers are undetermined. Foreign Ph.D. students have increased in the 1990s to the point where they make up 37 percent of biomedical research graduates and 17 percent of behavioral research graduates. A further increase in the number of foreign students could affect the workforce if it is not counterbalanced by a change in stay rates. If stay rates for foreign students decline, additional numbers of U.S. citizens and permanent residents could enter the workforce without increasing its overall size. Finally, our understanding of the health research workforce could be improved by incorporating clinical researchers into this analysis. Existing data on M.D.s and other doctoral-level health care professionals in research is insufficient to project the size of the clinical research workforce, but such an assessment might be undertaken with additional data collection and analysis.

[14] Ibid.

Three other transitions have been ignored, partly for reasons of data and partly because they appear inconsequential; however, this cannot be established with certainty. The first of these is emigration of Ph.D.s; only the emigration of foreign graduates who leave shortly after graduation has received attention. The second is return migration of these emigrant Ph.D.s. (There are a few return migrants among foreign graduates, as Finn's[15] data show, and there may be more among U.S.-born Ph.D.s.) The third is the return to the workforce of those who have retired. Introducing such transitions into the model could lead to a number of complications. It may be desirable, for instance, to determine a separate mortality schedule for the retired. The importance of considering such transitions in more detail depends on the precision required in projections and their potential uses. Nevertheless, such other transitions, and most of the specifications used here, would be better understood and modeled with more complete data.

TECHNICAL NOTE: THE PROJECTION MODEL

The projection model is illustrated in Figure D-1. It is a multistate life-table model, as recommended by a previous committee of the National Research Council,[16] but various specifics differ.

For any group specified by field and gender, the number employed in science at age j in year i is represented by E_{ji}, and similarly the number unemployed is U_{ji}, the number not in the labor force is V_{ji}, and the number outside science is O_{ji}. The potential workforce of the specified gender in a given field then is

$$W_{ji} = E_{ji} + U_{ji} + V_{ji}$$

with j running from age 25 to age 76.

Let the probability of moving from employment to unemployment from one year to the next at a given

[15] Finn, Michael G. "Stay Rates of Foreign Doctorate Recipients from U.S. Universities, 1995." Oak Ridge, Tenn.: Oak Ridge Institute for Science and Education, 1997.

[16] National Research Council. *The Use of Multi-State Life Tables in Estimating Places for Biomedical and Behavioral Scientists: A Technical Paper*. Washington, D.C.: National Academy Press, 1997.

starting age j be represented by eu_j, the probability of moving from employment out of the labor force by ev_j, the probability of moving from employment in science to outside science by eo_j, and the other probabilities of movement between these groups be similarly represented. Add the notation er_j to represent transition from being employed to being retired, and ed_j from being employed to being dead (and similarly for the other employment-status groups, but note that, given no better data, the mortality schedule is assumed to be identical across groups). These probabilities are all assumed to be constant over time.

The probabilities are also assumed to be conditional one on the next. For example, the probability of moving from employment to retirement is conditional on the individual's not dying in that period. Conditional probabilities are convenient to use because this simplifies the assumptions one has to make in estimating them from the data.

From these definitions, one can represent those at a given age j+1 who are employed in science in a given year i+1, leaving out new entrants, as

$$\begin{aligned} E_{j+1,i+1} = {} & E_{ji}\,(1\text{-}ed_j)\,(1\text{-}er_j)\,(1\text{-}ev_j)\,(1\text{-}eu_j)\,(1\text{-}eo_j) + \\ & U_{ji}\,(1\text{-}ud_j)\,(1\text{-}ur_j)\,(1\text{-}uv_j)\,(1\text{-}uo_j)ue_j + \\ & V_{ji}\,(1\text{-}vd_j)\,(1\text{-}vr_j)\,(1\text{-}vu_j)\,(1\text{-}vo_j)\,ve_j + \\ & O_{ji}\,(1\text{-}od_j)\,(1\text{-}or_j)\,(1\text{-}ov_j)\,(1\text{-}ou_j)\,oe_j. \end{aligned}$$

Similar expressions apply to the other employment status groups.

Graduates (G_{ji}) and immigrants (H_{ji}) entering the workforce at age j in year i are projected as discussed in the text. For graduates, the specific equations on year since 1900 ($y = i - 1900$) for the high projection are as follows:

Male biomedical scientists
$12{,}438 - 307\,y + 2.18\,y^2$, $R^2 = 0.98$
Female biomedical scientists
$20{,}178 - 515\,y + 3.42\,y^2$, $R^2 = 0.99$
Male behavioral scientists
$26{,}930 - 557\,y + 2.99\,y^2$, $R^2 = 0.84$
Female behavioral scientists
$10{,}071 - 221\,y + 1.37\,y^2$, $R^2 = 0.87$

For behavioral scientists, the equations for the low projection are

Male behavioral scientists
$4{,}313 - 29\,y - 0.07\,y^2$, $R^2 = 0.86$
Female behavioral scientists
$-10{,}718 + 256\,y + 1.35\,y^2$, $R^2 = 0.93$

For biomedical scientists the low projection is based on a constant number of graduates. For all groups the medium projection is the average of the high and the low projections.

Graduates who stay in the country and immigrants are assumed to distribute themselves across the four employment status groups (including outside science) in proportion to those already in these groups at age j in year i. In case there are fewer than 50 individuals already at a given age, proportions are taken over three or five contiguous single-year age groups and, if this criterion is still not met, over the entire age distribution. Entering graduates and immigrants are assumed not to retire or die for at least a year. Graduates are limited to the age range 25-50 and immigrants to the age range 25-70.

To estimate the number of entering graduates necessary to keep the total workforce constant over time, a projection is run one year at a time assuming no graduates. The gap between the projected workforce and the starting workforce is then estimated, and the graduates necessary to fill this gap are calculated, which allows this number to be greater than the actual gap because some graduates leave the country and others take jobs outside science.

These graduates can be distributed by age to parallel their distribution in the year before the projection starts. Designate this year as year 0 and let pw_j stand for the proportion in the workforce (as opposed to outside science) at age j. Then

$$G_{ji} = \frac{G_{j0}\,3_j(kW_{j0} - W_{ji})}{3_j G_{j0} pw_j},$$

where $k = 1$. To allow the workforce to grow or decline by some fixed rate, k can be set equal to one plus that rate.

The projections require Ph.D. immigrants by year, which are estimated by reverse survival. The first step is to divide the two-year cohorts in the survey arbitrarily in half to give single-year cohorts and facilitate calculations. The number of migrants resident in the U.S. is assumed to be equal to the number entering the country, after adjustment for retirement and death over the period since entry. (Other transitions, such as return migration, are not considered.) For age group j, let R_{ji} represent the immigrants remaining in the country in year i. Also define s_j as the survival rate for age group j, the proportion that neither die nor retire in one year:

$$s_j = (1 - td_j)\,(1 - tr_j),$$

where td_j is the weighted proportion dying among those employed, unemployed, not in the labor force, and outside science (= ed_j, the proportions for all these groups being equal), and tr_j is the weighted proportion retiring among those in these groups who do not die. (These factors are specific by field and gender, but subscripts are not shown for that.) Then the immigrants entering in 1985-86 should be

$$R_{j,1985.5} = R_{j+8,1993} / s_{j-1} / s_{j-2} / s_{j-3} / s_{j-4} / s_{j-5} / s_{j-6} / s_{j-7} / / s_{j-8}$$

The results of these calculations were converted to annual numbers, dividing each two-year period in two. Figures for the last period (1987-90) were divided by 3.5, on the assumption that the period is truncated because migration had to take place before the 1990 census. After averaging across periods, the distribution by age was smoothed using five-year moving averages.

Appendix E

Classification of Ph.D. Fields

BASIC BIOMEDICAL SCIENCES

Anatomy
Bacteriology
Biochemistry
Biological Immunology
Biological Sciences, General
Biological Sciences, Other
Biomedical Engineering
Biomedical Sciences
Biophysics
Biotechnology Research
Cell Biology
Developmental Biology/Embryology
Endocrinology
Genetics, Human and Animal
Medicinal/Pharmaceutical Chemistry
Microbiology
Molecular Biology
Neuroscience
Nutritional Sciences
Parasitology
Pathology, Human and Animal
Pharmacology, Human and Animal
Physiology
Toxicology
Veterinary Medicine
Zoology

CLINICAL SCIENCES

Biometrics and Biostatistics
Environmental Health
Epidemiology
Exercise Physiology/Science
Health Sciences, General
Health Sciences, Other
Health Systems/Services Administration
Nursing
Pharmacy
Public Health
Rehabilitation/Therapeutic Services

BEHAVIORAL AND SOCIAL SCIENCES

Anthropology
Audiology and Speech Pathology
Demography/Population Studies
Sociology

Psychology

Cognitive and Psycholinguistics
Comparative
Developmental and Child
Educational
Experimental
Industrial and Organizational
Personality
Psychology, General
Psychology, Other
Psychometrics
Physiological/Psychobiology
Quantitative
Social

NOTE: These are fields in which Ph.D.s are awarded, as classified by the Survey of Earned Doctorates, the annual census of doctoral recipients from U.S. universities that has been conducted from 1920 to the present. The same field names are used in the Survey of Doctoral Recipients, the biennial workforce survey of U.S. science and engineering Ph.D.s. Analyses of Ph.D. production and the employment patterns of biomedical, behavioral, and clinical scientists conducted for this report also incorporated field names comparable to those identified here but no longer in use (e.g., the combined field of microbiology and bacteriology, which was eliminated in 1983 and replaced by the two distinct fields listed above).

Appendix F

Personal Statement Concerning Research Training in the Behavioral and Social Sciences

John F. Kihlstrom
University of California, Berkeley

I generally agree with the findings, conclusions, and recommendations of the Committee on National Needs for Biomedical and Behavioral Scientists. I believe, however, that the committee has not fully considered the actual and potential contributions that the behavioral and social sciences can make to health and health care and the implications of these contributions for the National Research Service Award (NRSA) training program and related training activities sponsored by the National Institutes of Health, the Agency for Healthcare Research and Quality, and the Health Resources and Services Administration. In this "personal statement" I wish to outline briefly some of these contributions and some of their implications for training.

CONTRIBUTIONS OF THE BEHAVIORAL AND SOCIAL SCIENCES TO HEALTH AND HEALTH CARE

Behavioral and social factors play a central role in health and illness. A widely cited study found that more than half of premature deaths in the United States during 1990 could be attributed directly to behavioral and social factors, including tobacco use, diet and activity patterns, alcohol, firearms, sexual practices, the operation of motor vehicles, and drug use.[1] Taken together, tobacco use, diet, and activity accounted for approximately five times as many premature deaths as did microbial and toxic agents. Similar findings are contained in periodic analyses of the leading causes of death published by the Centers for Disease Control and Prevention. In addition, the study cited evidence that problems of access to primary care, screening, and preventive care accounted for approximately 7 percent of premature deaths and that poverty has a direct effect on mortality, independent of access to care. In fact, socioeconomic status is one of the most reliable predictors of both health and longevity.

The case of HIV/AIDS offers dramatic testimony to the role that the behavioral and social sciences can play in health and illness. Almost two decades after the identification of AIDS (in 1981) and the isolation of the HIV virus (in 1983) and extensive biomedical research, there is still no cure and no vaccine. Nevertheless, psychosocial interventions, taking account of both the determinants of individual behavior and the wider sociocultural context in which individual behavior takes place have effectively reduced the incidence of HIV-related sexual risk behaviors.[2] According to Thomas J. Coates and Chris Collins, "altering behavior" through targeted education, peer influence and community action, advertising, and marketing remains "the primary way to control the epidemic" of HIV-AIDS.[3] An NIH Consensus Development Conference Statement, prepared by a nonadvocate nonfederal panel of experts, concluded that "behavioral interventions to reduce risk

[1] McGinnis, J. Michael, and William H. Foege. "Actual Causes of Death in the United States." *JAMA*, 270(1993): 2207-12.

[2] National Institute of Mental Health (NIMH) Multisite HIV Prevention Trial Group. "The NIMH Multisite HIV Prevention Trial: Reducing HIV Sexual Risk Behavior." *Science* 280(1998):1889-94.

[3] Coates, Thomas J., and Chris Collins. "Preventing HIV Infection." *Scientific American* (July 1998): 96-97.

for HIV/AIDS are effective and should be disseminated widely."[4]

Although some drug treatments (such as AZT) have been developed that greatly slow the progression of HIV to AIDS, compliance with these treatments by HIV-infected individuals is often remarkably poor given what is at stake. In fact, across a wide variety of chronic and life-threatening diseases, from asthma and hypertension to epilepsy and renal disease, compliance with prescribed medical regimens is universally acknowledged to be a central problem for health care professionals. According to some analyses, as many as 50 percent or more of patients take prescribed medicines improperly—if they take them at all. The situation is just as bad, if not worse, for compliance with such disease prevention regimes as diet and exercise. The problem of compliance underscores the fact that developing a pill is only one step toward effective treatment or prevention. We must also get patients to take their pills: This is a behavioral problem that must be addressed at the individual and sociocultural levels of analysis.

It is now understood that stress (including job stress and burnout) and negative emotionality are important risk factors for disease, while social support and positive emotionality are significant factors in reducing both morbidity and mortality. While the bacterium *h. pylori* is found in the intestinal tracts of most if not all individuals suffering from ulcers, not everyone infected with *h. pylori* gets an ulcer: According to one theory, stress levels make the difference between health and disease. Although some of the neuroendocrine and neuroimmunological mechanisms underlying "psychosomatic" relationships are becoming known, the fact remains that both stress and social support are properly defined in psychosocial rather than physiological terms. Certain environments are more stressful than others, and in the final analysis it is the individual's mental representation of these environments that arouses stress. Although biological interventions may be able to alter the body's response to stress, the key(s) to alleviating stress itself will be found at the individual and social levels.

The psychosocial aspects of health encompass not just health and disease but a wide variety of health behaviors, broadly defined. The maintenance of health and the prevention of disease require individuals to engage in healthy behaviors, consult health care professionals when they experience the symptoms of disease, and participate actively in both the treatment of acute illnesses and rehabilitation of chronic disease. Somatization disorder, and the inappropriate and expensive use of health services that it entails, remains one of the most vexing mental health problems encountered in primary care and general hospital practice. The adverse health consequences of tobacco use are best prevented by convincing people not to smoke in the first place. The prognosis of breast cancer is best with early detection through a program of regular self-examination and appropriate mammograms. Proper treatment of hypertension requires that an individual take prescribed drugs even though he or she will not experience any relief of subjective symptoms. Successful management of renal disease is not accomplished by transplant or dialysis alone: In either case the patient must also make significant lifestyle changes. Health behavior, illness behavior, the sick role, and rehabilitation are not matters of anatomy and physiology: They are matters of behavior, society, and culture. They require coordinated and integrated attack by behavioral and social scientists working across the disciplines—and especially by investigators whose approaches transcend the boundaries of the traditional disciplines.

We have seen radical changes in the organization of health care, including changes in the duties of established professions such as pharmacy; the proliferation of new professions (such as nurse practitioners and physician assistants) involved in primary care; the impact of third-party payments on the practice of medicine; the rise of evidence-based medicine and other aspects of "managed" care; the "carving up" of health care through disease management and other programs; the advertising of pharmaceuticals directly to patients; the increasing acceptance of dietary supplements, herbal remedies, and other alternatives to traditional medications; and the availability of vast amounts of medical information, of variable quality, over the Internet. The advent of managed care creates at least the appearance of conflict between the ethical responsibilities of doctors to their patients and their financial responsibilities to their families and their employers. Physicians, once largely private practitioners, are increasingly cast in the role of employees: They have even begun to unionize. Health care, once a matter of a private relationship between doctor and patient, practiced in private offices and hospital wards, is now an

[4] "Interventions to Prevent HIV Risk Behaviors." NIH Consensus Development Program, vol. 15, no. 2, February 11-13, 1997. The full consensus statement is available at http://odp.od.nih.gov/consensus/cons/104/104.htm.

extremely complex and often mysterious industry. All these trends have irrevocably changed the relationships between health care providers and consumers, among providers, and between providers and payers. Understanding and coping with these changes is a matter for the social sciences; and none of the traditional disciplines operating alone is adequate to the task.

The United States is an increasingly diverse and multicultural society. Once portrayed by John Dewey as a great melting pot, American society is increasingly being recognized as a stew, in which each individual ingredient retains its identity. Nathan Glazer, whose *Beyond the Melting Pot* is a classic study of the immigrant experience,[5] has concluded in his most recent book that *We Are All Multiculturalists Now*.[6] The health and illness behavior of "new Americans" may be determined to a large extent by their cultural background and the conceptions(s) of health and illness that flow from it. Nowhere is this better illustrated than in Anne Fadiman's book, *The Spirit Catches You and You Fall Down*,[7] which portrays the conflict between traditional Hmong culture and advanced Western medicine in the treatment of the infant Lia Lee, daughter of Laotian immigrants living in Merced County, California. Lia's doctors diagnosed epilepsy and prescribed anticonvulsant drugs, while her parents ascribed her condition to a wandering soul *(qaug dab peg)* and wanted to perform animal sacrifices. Although most health care episodes may not entail such a dramatic conflict of cultures, the point remains that, in twenty-first-century American society, effective strategies for the prevention and treatment of disease require that health care providers be sensitive to cultural differences that may exist between their patients and themselves.

BEHAVIORAL AND SOCIAL SCIENCE TRAINING AT THE NATIONAL INSTITUTES OF HEALTH

Considerations such as these suggest that the behavioral and social sciences are just as much basic sciences for health as the traditional "biomedical" fields are. Nevertheless, it appears that the NIH investment in NRSA research training in the behavioral and social sciences is not commensurate with the contributions that they have to offer the health care enterprise.

As just one example, Tables G-7 and G-8 of the committee's report indicate that, during 1997, NIH and other Department of Health and Human Services (DHHS) traineeships and fellowships were the primary source of financial support for 11.6 percent (3,941 out of 33,873) of graduate students in the basic biomedical sciences but only 2.3 percent (563 out of 24,988) of graduate students in the behavioral and social sciences. In fact, these tables show that over the entire period 1975-1997, DHHS traineeship and fellowship support for students in the behavioral and social sciences declined from 19.1 percent in 1975 to 2.3 percent in 1997; HHS training grant and fellowship support for students in the biomedical sciences declined as well, but less severely: from 24.7 percent in 1975 to 11.6 percent in 1997. Of course, as the committee's report notes, not all behavioral and social science graduate students are engaged in health-related research, while (almost by definition) virtually all biomedical science graduate students do so. Still, it seems unlikely that the drop in traineeship and fellowship support in the behavioral and social sciences was accompanied by a decrease in the numbers of careers in health research available for these students. In any case, the discrepancy suggests that NIH policies should more aggressively encourage graduate students in the behavioral and social sciences to focus their efforts on problems more closely related to health and health care. Certainly that was the recommendation of the previous incarnation of this committee, which in 1994 recommended that the number of NRSA awards for pre- and postdoctoral research training in the behavioral and social sciences increase 35 percent by 1996, while maintaining the basic biomedical sciences at their 1993 levels. The U.S. Congress seconded this recommendation, and beginning in 1995 it has continuously requested that the NIH develop and execute a plan to implement it. While the number of NIH and DHHS traineeships and fellowships in the basic biomedical sciences did indeed hold constant between 1993 and 1997 (4,001 and 3,941 recipients, respectively, according to Table G-7 of the committee's report), the number in the behavioral and social sciences increased only about 4 percent, from 539 to 563 (Table G-8).

As important as the sheer amount of support is, it is also important to understand where that support comes from and where it is going. Table F-1 summarizes an analysis of the sources of NRSA funding for Ph.D. re-

[5] Glazer, Nathan, and Daniel P. Moynihan. *Beyond the Melting Pot.* Cambridge, Mass.: MIT Press.

[6] Glazer, Nathan. *We Are All Multiculturalists Now.* Cambridge, Mass.: Harvard University Press, 1997.

[7] Fadiman, Anne. *The Spirit Catches You and You Fall Down: A Hmong Child, Her American Doctors, and the Collision of Two Cultures.* New York: Farrar, Straus, & Giroux, 1998.

TABLE F-1 Sources of Predoctoral NRSA Research Training Support for 1995 Ph.D. Recipients in the Biomedical and Behavioral Sciences

Source	All Biomedical	Anthropology	Demography	Economics	Psychology	Sociology	Speech Pathology
Agency for Healthcare Research and Quality	0	0	0	1	0	0	0
National Institute on Alcohol Abuse and Alcoholism	6	0	0	0	4	0	0
National Institute on Aging	11	0	1	0	12	9	1
National Institute of Allergy and Infectious Diseases	65	0	0	0	0	0	0
National Institute of Arthritis and Musculoskeletal and Skin Diseases	3	0	0	0	0	0	0
National Cancer Institute	132	1	0	0	0	0	0
National Institute on Drug Abuse	12	0	0	0	8	1	0
National Institute on Deafness and Other Communication Disorders	3	0		0	2	0	2
National Institute of Dental and Craniofacial Research	4	0	0	0	3	0	0
National Institute of Diabetes and Digestive and Kidney Diseases	16	0	0	0	0	0	0
National Institute of Environmental Health Sciences	57	0	0	0	0	0	0
National Eye Institute	24	0	0	0	1	0	0
National Institute of General Medical Sciences	675	0	0	0	2	2	0
National Institute of Child Health and Human Development	47	1	4	0	27	14	0
National Human Genome Research Institute	3	0	0	0	0	0	0
National Heart, Lung, and Blood Institute	57	0	0	0	9	0	0
National Institute of Mental Health	50	7	0	0	107	11	0
National Institute of Nursing Research	2	0	0	0	1	0	0
National Institute of Neurological Disorders and Stroke	27	0	0	0	0	0	0

SOURCES: Data are from the NIH Trainee and Fellow File and the Survey of Earned Doctorates.

cipients in the biomedical and behavioral sciences in 1995 who received funding from the NRSA program during graduate school.[8] According to this information, federal agencies and NIH institutes provided NRSA training support to 1,194 individuals who received Ph.D.s in the biomedical sciences (83.8 percent of the biomedical and behavioral Ph.D.s who received NRSA funding) and 231 individuals who received Ph.D.s in the behavioral and social sciences (16.2 percent of those with NRSA funding) that year. The table shows the agency or institute that provided the NRSA support and, within the behavioral and social sciences, the particular discipline in which individuals received their Ph.D.s (individuals who received their Ph.D.s in health services research and other "clinical research disciplines" are not included in the analysis).

Within NIH, responsibility for training in the behavioral and social sciences has fallen mostly to the three institutes formerly under the umbrella of the Alcohol, Drug Abuse, and Mental Health Administration (ADAMHA): the National Institute on Alcohol Abuse and Alcoholism (NIAAA), National Institute on Drug Abuse (NIDA), and National Institute of Mental Health

[8] Based on Tables 4 and 5 attached to a fax distributed to the committee on 7/10/98.

(NIMH). Of the 231 Ph.D.s in the behavioral and social sciences who had received NRSA funding in graduate school, 125 (54.1 percent) were supported by NIMH and an additional 4 (1.7 percent) and 9 (3.9 percent) by NIAAA and NIDA, respectively, accounting for 59.7 percent of the total with NRSA support. The National Institute of Child Health and Human Development (NICHD) accounted for 46 individuals (19.9 percent) and the National Institute on Aging (NIA) for 23 individuals (10 percent). Not surprisingly, the one individual supported by the Agency for Health Care Policy and Research (AHCPR; now the Agency for Healthcare Research and Quality) was in the behavioral and social sciences (in fact, the sole economist to receive predoctoral support through the NRSA program). The remaining 23 individuals (10 percent of the total) were distributed over the remaining 11 NIH institutes.

Closer inspection of Table F-1 reveals that the distribution of biomedical and behavioral science Ph.D.s varies greatly from institute to institute. Of the 206 Ph.D. recipients in 1995 who were supported by NRSA awards through the former ADAMHA institutes, 138 (67 percent) were in the behavioral and social sciences, compared to 68 (33 percent) in the biomedical sciences. For NIA and NICHD, the behavioral and social sciences accounted for 67.7 percent and 49.5 percent of their 34 and 93 recipients, respectively (as noted earlier, the one recipient from AHCPR was in a behavioral and social science discipline). For the remaining 11 NIH institutes, the percentages are dramatically reversed: only 2.2 percent of the 1,092 Ph.D. recipients in 1995 were in the behavioral and social sciences. For example, even though the behavioral and social sciences are basic sciences for health, the basic biomedical sciences accounted for 99.4 percent of recipients supported by the National Institute of General Medical Sciences (NIGMS). Despite considerable advances in behavior genetics, not a single Ph.D. in the behavioral and social sciences was supported by the National Human Genome Research Institute.

Almost all the predoctoral research training provided in the behavioral and social sciences goes to psychologists. As indicated in Table F-1, psychologists accounted for 176 (76.2 percent), and sociologists for an additional 37 (16 percent), with 18 individuals divided among anthropology, demography, economics, and speech pathology. Psychologists supported by NIMH accounted for 107 individuals, or 46.3 percent of the total recipients of NRSA funding in the behavioral and social sciences.

Given the central role that the behavioral and social sciences have played, historically, in understanding and treating mental illness and substance abuse, it is not surprising that the training activities of the former ADAMHA institutes are rather heavily weighted in their direction. However, in view of the contributions that the behavioral and social sciences can and do make to the health care enterprise, it is rather disconcerting to learn that the remaining institutes have devoted so few resources to training in these fields.

ALTERNATIVE RECOMMENDATIONS

The committee majority has chosen not to repeat or reinforce its predecessor's call for increases in NRSA awards in the behavioral and social sciences and, indeed, has recommended that there should be no growth in the annual number of doctorates awarded in these fields. In view of the apparent underemployment of behavioral and social science Ph.D.s, and the possible overproduction of Ph.D.s in some specialties, it is hard to gainsay this latter recommendation. I believe, however, that the committee should have taken the opportunity to recommend policies that would redirect more current and future students in these fields into research training more directly related to health and health care. With the establishment of the Office of Behavioral and Social Science Research, NIH has taken an important step forward in recognizing the contributions of the behavioral and social sciences to health and health care and in promoting these fields within the institutes. But our committee is particularly concerned with research training, and in this respect it seems clear that NIH and DHHS can and should do more.

1. The NIH and DHHS should expand their training activities in the behavioral and social sciences, especially as they pertain to health and health behavior, without reducing the amount of behavioral and social science training supported by the former ADAMHA institutes and other institutes that are already doing a great deal in this direction. That is to say, the current level of behavioral and social science training supported by NRSA should not merely be spread more broadly over the NIH institutes. Rather, new funds should be provided so that all institutes can support their fair share of behavioral and social sciences research training, without compromising the training ac-

tivities already on the books at such institutes as NIMH and NICHD.

2. What is the meaning of "fair share"? Although the behavioral and social sciences are relevant to the mission of each of the NIH institutes, the institutes vary widely in terms of the amount of funding devoted to research training in these disciplines. According to figures developed by the Center for the Advancement of Health, some NIH institutes devoted almost a third of their 1998 training budgets to the behavioral and social sciences, while other institutes devoted less than 1 percent; the median value was approximately 7 percent.[9] As a first step, new funds earmarked for training in the behavioral and social sciences should be provided to those institutes whose current support in this area is minimal. As a second step, additional new funds should be allocated to those institutes that already make substantial contributions to training in the behavioral and social sciences, in order to permit them to expand their efforts in this area. The intent of this recommendation is to enable NIH institutes to expand their training efforts in the behavioral and social sciences without requiring a reallocation of existing funds, which would compromise efforts already underway. It would be a mistake for those institutes that now provide the bulk of behavioral and social science support to reduce their efforts in these areas. But the NIMH, NIA, and NICHHD should not be expected to carry the weight of behavioral and social science research training for the entire NIH. In particular, the National Institute of General Medical Sciences should increase its training efforts in the behavioral and social sciences in recognition of the fact that these fields are as much "basic sciences" for health as are anatomy and physiology.

3. Each of the NIH institutes should ensure that its training portfolio includes diverse representation from the disciplines constituting the behavioral and social sciences. As things currently stand, the vast bulk of training funds in the behavioral and social sciences goes to psychology. Training funds should not be diverted away from psychology to cover other behavioral and social sciences. All the disciplines have important contributions to make. Instead, the expansion of research training in the behavioral and social sciences should be supported by the new funds recommended above.

4. The preceding analysis and recommendations have been couched in terms of the traditional behavioral and social science disciplines, such as anthropology, psychology, and sociology, because that is the way data analyses have been presented to the committee. In the future, however, it seems likely that the most important contributions of the behavioral and social sciences to health and health care will be made by interdisciplinary fields such as health services research, which approach problems from several different angles. Such interdisciplinary efforts are likely to contribute more to health and health care than any single discipline, such as psychology, can do. The committee is right to call for special attention to interdisciplinary research. The text of the recommendation, however, implies that these interdisciplinary activities will likely involve the brain sciences and medicine. It should be understood that the behavioral and social sciences are full sciences in their own right, and interdisciplinary efforts by scientists in these fields can proceed independently of neuroscience, behavior genetics, and other fields of biology.

5. Although the committee's report and this addendum have focused on NRSA support for research training support specifically related to health, it should be understood that basic research in the behavioral and social sciences, no less than basic research in the physical and biological sciences, lays the foundation for health-related research. It goes without saying that the development of brain-imaging techniques relies on basic research in physics and the development of new pharmaceuticals relies on basic research in biochemistry. In exactly the same way, understanding the problem of medication compliance relies on basic research on the nature of beliefs and attitudes; understanding the health care recommendations and choices of providers, patients, and payees relies on basic research on human judgment and decision-making processes; understanding the changing relations among stakeholders in the health care system relies on basic research on organizational structures and behavior; and understanding ethnic differences in health and illness behavior relies on basic research on the nature of culture. While it is understandable that the various NIH institutes would prefer to support behavioral and social science training that is specifically targeted toward their unique missions, each individual institute should be asked to support a mix of basic and applied research training.

[9] Center for the Advancement of Health. *Cultivating Capacity: Advancing NIH Research Training in the Health-Related Behavior and Social Sciences.* Washington, D.C.: Center for the Advancement of Health, 1999.

Just as effective research on health and health care will require that we transcend the boundaries of the various disciplines, so it will require that we tear down the wall that divides the basic from the applied.

6. Allocation of additional funds for research training in the behavioral and social sciences will not have its intended effect unless academic institutions apply for them, and academic institutions will not apply for training support unless there is a reasonable chance of success. Accordingly, each of the NIH institutes and DHHS agencies should issue Requests for Applications for behavioral and social science training relevant to their missions. Moreover, the Center for Scientific Review (formerly the Division of Research Grants) should ensure that its system of review panels contains sufficient numbers of behavioral and social scientists to ensure that these applications will receive expert and sympathetic review.

Appendix G

Supplementary Tables

TABLE G-1 Demographic Characteristics of Ph.D. Recipients in the Basic Biomedical Sciences

	1975	1976	1977	1978	1979	1980	1981	1982	1983	1984
Total	3085 100.0%	3150 100.0%	3050 100.0%	3118 100.0%	3212 100.0%	3396 100.0%	3356 100.0%	3444 100.0%	3338 100.0%	3399 100.0%
Men	2347 76.1%	2424 77.0%	2351 77.1%	2311 74.1%	2351 73.2%	2440 71.8%	2383 71.0%	2417 70.2%	2224 66.6%	2315 68.1%
Women	738 23.9%	726 23.0%	699 22.9%	807 25.9%	861 26.8%	956 28.2%	973 29.0%	1027 29.8%	1114 33.4%	1084 31.9%
Minorities[a]	74 2.4%	72 2.3%	58 1.9%	87 2.8%	67 2.1%	75 2.2%	91 2.7%	94 2.7%	86 2.6%	98 2.9%
U.S. citizens	2554 82.8%	2609 82.8%	2525 82.8%	2626 84.2%	2738 85.2%	2904 85.5%	2897 86.3%	2919 84.8%	2850 85.4%	2866 84.3%
Permanent residents	194 6.3%	165 5.2%	169 5.5%	147 4.7%	133 4.1%	147 4.3%	125 3.7%	114 3.3%	108 3.2%	109 3.2%
Temporary visas	256 8.3%	277 8.8%	261 8.6%	259 8.3%	253 7.9%	273 8.0%	248 7.4%	294 8.5%	291 8.7%	308 9.1%
Planning postdoctoral study	1891 61.3%	1937 61.5%	1966 64.5%	2086 66.9%	2127 66.2%	2316 68.2%	2305 68.7%	2363 68.6%	2298 68.8%	2377 69.9%
Median time to Ph.D. (in years)[b]	6.00	6.17	6.25	6.33	6.41	6.50	6.50	6.67	7.00	7.09
Median age at tme of degree	29.25	29.25	29.34	29.38	29.41	29.25	29.33	29.59	29.83	30.25

[a] African Americans, Hispanics, and Native Americans; tabulations include U.S. citizens and permanent residents only.
[b] From entry into graduate studies.

SOURCE: Data are from the Survey of Earned Doctorates.

1985	1986	1987	1988	1989	1990	1991	1992	1993	1994	1995	1996	1997
3313	3369	3465	3769	3793	3992	4309	4456	4823	4881	5101	5385	5420
100.0%	100.0%	100.0%	100.0%	100.0%	100.0%	100.0%	100.0%	100.0%	100.0%	100.0%	100.0%	100.0%
2192	2197	2214	2377	2348	2477	2655	2740	2864	2887	2955	3101	3069
66.2%	65.2%	63.9%	63.1%	61.9%	62.0%	61.6%	61.5%	59.4%	59.1%	57.9%	57.6%	56.6%
1121	1172	1251	1392	1445	1515	1639	1702	1930	1976	2125	2264	2319
33.8%	34.8%	36.1%	36.9%	38.1%	38.0%	38.0%	38.2%	40.0%	40.5%	41.7%	42.0%	42.8%
104	118	127	122	133	135	159	161	183	220	236	240	255
3.1%	3.5%	3.7%	3.2%	3.5%	3.4%	3.7%	3.6%	3.8%	4.5%	4.6%	4.5%	4.7%
2725	2751	2670	2858	2850	2899	3050	3072	3264	3203	3278	3291	3415
82.3%	81.7%	77.1%	75.8%	75.1%	72.6%	70.8%	68.9%	67.7%	65.6%	64.3%	61.1%	63.0%
113	118	153	176	173	183	210	240	296	641	831	801	553
3.4%	3.5%	4.4%	4.7%	4.6%	4.6%	4.9%	5.4%	6.1%	13.1%	16.3%	14.9%	10.2%
364	343	455	515	570	814	987	1078	1165	980	919	1172	1170
11.0%	10.2%	13.1%	13.7%	15.0%	20.4%	22.9%	24.2%	24.2%	20.1%	18.0%	21.8%	21.6%
2309	2368	2419	2651	2656	2886	3160	3293	3614	3626	3806	3931	3529
69.7%	70.3%	69.8%	70.3%	70.0%	72.3%	73.3%	73.9%	74.9%	74.3%	74.6%	73.0%	65.1%
7.17	7.25	7.33	7.42	7.42	7.58	7.50	7.59	7.67	7.75	7.83	7.67	7.83
30.42	30.59	30.50	30.83	30.92	31.17	31.08	31.17	31.17	31.17	31.25	31.25	30.92

TABLE G-2 Demographic Characteristics of Ph.D. Recipients in the Behavioral and Social Sciences

	1975	1976	1977	1978	1979	1980	1981	1982	1983	1984
Total	2794	2897	2893	2743	2736	2610	2729	2507	2590	2482
	100.0%	100.0%	100.0%	100.0%	100.0%	100.0%	100.0%	100.0%	100.0%	100.0%
Men	1899	1949	1860	1725	1623	1535	1568	1397	1385	1256
	68.0%	67.3%	64.3%	62.9%	59.3%	58.8%	57.5%	55.7%	53.5%	50.6%
Women	895	948	1033	1018	1113	1075	1161	1110	1205	1226
	32.0%	32.7%	35.7%	37.1%	40.7%	41.2%	42.5%	44.3%	46.5%	49.4%
Minorities[a]	114	130	129	139	157	149	141	158	147	144
	4.1%	4.5%	4.5%	5.1%	5.7%	5.7%	5.2%	6.3%	5.7%	5.8%
U.S. citizens	2464	2598	2554	2448	2440	2301	2389	2157	2220	2100
	88.2%	89.7%	88.3%	89.2%	89.2%	88.2%	87.5%	86.0%	85.7%	84.6%
Permanent residents	75	76	81	79	79	86	68	66	67	49
	2.7%	2.6%	2.8%	2.9%	2.9%	3.3%	2.5%	2.6%	2.6%	2.0%
Temporary visas	190	168	154	133	147	138	150	131	163	177
	6.8%	5.8%	5.3%	4.8%	5.4%	5.3%	5.5%	5.2%	6.3%	7.1%
Planning postdoctoral study	349	392	441	480	444	459	465	409	469	444
	12.5%	13.5%	15.2%	17.5%	16.2%	17.6%	17.0%	16.3%	18.1%	17.9%
Median time to Ph.D. (in years)[b]	6.25	6.33	6.59	6.92	7.17	7.33	7.63	8.00	8.00	8.25
Median age at time of degree	30.42	30.58	30.83	30.83	31.42	31.75	32.08	32.34	32.75	33.00

[a] African Americans, Hispanics, and Native Americans; tabulations include U.S. citizens and permanent residents only.
[b] From entry into graduate studies.

SOURCE: Data are from the Survey of Earned Doctorates.

1985	1986	1987	1988	1989	1990	1991	1992	1993	1994	1995	1996	1997
2352	2357	2288	2268	2215	2261	2290	2273	2439	2411	2406	2434	2591
100.0%	100.0%	100.0%	100.0%	100.0%	100.0%	100.0%	100.0%	100.0%	100.0%	100.0%	100.0%	100.0%
1187	1180	1133	1046	1030	1008	977	1031	1019	1042	1013	982	1012
50.5%	50.1%	49.5%	46.1%	46.5%	44.6%	42.7%	45.4%	41.8%	43.2%	42.1%	40.3%	39.1%
1165	1177	1155	1222	1185	1253	1309	1236	1412	1362	1388	1444	1558
49.5%	49.9%	50.5%	53.9%	53.5%	55.4%	57.2%	54.4%	57.9%	56.5%	57.7%	59.3%	60.1%
152	144	126	147	139	169	182	157	183	188	221	200	219
6.5%	6.1%	5.5%	6.5%	6.3%	7.5%	7.9%	6.9%	7.5%	7.8%	9.2%	8.2%	8.5%
1975	1936	1819	1807	1684	1851	1869	1812	1964	1944	1915	1943	1927
84.0%	82.1%	79.5%	79.7%	76.0%	81.9%	81.6%	79.7%	80.5%	80.6%	79.6%	79.8%	74.4%
72	77	87	74	70	72	97	94	104	128	137	137	117
3.1%	3.3%	3.8%	3.3%	3.2%	3.2%	4.2%	4.1%	4.3%	5.3%	5.7%	5.6%	4.5%
164	163	153	172	222	235	267	294	301	283	276	263	253
7.0%	6.9%	6.7%	7.6%	10.0%	10.4%	11.7%	12.9%	12.3%	11.7%	11.5%	10.8%	9.8%
434	493	459	459	406	438	495	488	532	555	567	521	486
18.5%	20.9%	20.1%	20.2%	18.3%	19.4%	21.6%	21.5%	21.8%	23.0%	23.6%	21.4%	18.8%
8.59	8.91	8.92	9.00	9.00	9.00	9.08	9.08	9.00	9.00	9.00	8.92	8.83
33.42	34.00	34.33	35.00	34.75	34.67	35.00	34.83	34.92	34.34	34.50	33.91	33.38

TABLE G-3 Demographic Characteristics of Ph.D. Recipients in the Clinical Sciences

	1975	1976	1977	1978	1979	1980	1981	1982	1983	1984
Total	230	241	276	289	311	337	367	416	526	621
	100.0%	100.0%	100.0%	100.0%	100.0%	100.0%	100.0%	100.0%	100.0%	100.0%
Men	158	176	196	208	202	204	221	232	249	262
	68.7%	73.0%	71.0%	72.0%	65.0%	60.5%	60.2%	55.8%	47.3%	42.2%
Women	72	65	80	81	109	133	146	184	277	359
	31.3%	27.0%	29.0%	28.0%	35.0%	39.5%	39.8%	44.2%	52.7%	57.8%
Minorities[a]	2	4	10	8	12	8	13	19	23	34
	0.9%	1.7%	3.6%	2.8%	3.9%	2.4%	3.5%	4.6%	4.4%	5.5%
U.S. citizens	171	181	213	223	240	256	292	328	401	492
	74.3%	75.1%	77.2%	77.2%	77.2%	76.0%	79.6%	78.8%	76.2%	79.2%
Permanent residents	31	27	34	23	32	27	29	25	30	36
	13.5%	11.2%	12.3%	8.0%	10.3%	8.0%	7.9%	6.0%	5.7%	5.8%
Temporary visas	21	28	25	28	27	45	34	48	70	66
	9.1%	11.6%	9.1%	9.7%	8.7%	13.4%	9.3%	11.5%	13.3%	10.6%
Planning postdoctoral study	43	51	64	57	78	87	81	84	69	104
	18.7%	21.2%	23.2%	19.7%	25.1%	25.8%	22.1%	20.2%	13.1%	16.7%
Median time to Ph.D. (in years)[b]	7.00	6.63	6.50	7.09	6.92	7.17	7.67	7.50	7.92	8.17
Median age at time of degree	31.83	31.58	30.79	31.67	31.75	32.00	32.37	32.87	34.08	34.33

[a] African Americans, Hispanics, and Native Americans; tabulations include U.S. citizens and permanent residents only.
[b] From entry into graduate studies.

SOURCE: Data are from the Survey of Earned Doctorates.

1985	1986	1987	1988	1989	1990	1991	1992	1993	1994	1995	1996	1997
619	677	699	788	881	840	954	1030	1112	1217	1236	1246	1349
100.0%	100.0%	100.0%	100.0%	100.0%	100.0%	100.0%	100.0%	100.0%	100.0%	100.0%	100.0%	100.0%
244	259	290	302	313	322	333	363	396	420	456	434	462
39.4%	38.3%	41.5%	38.3%	35.5%	38.3%	34.9%	35.2%	35.6%	34.5%	36.9%	34.8%	34.2%
375	418	409	486	568	518	617	659	704	787	769	803	870
60.6%	61.7%	58.5%	61.7%	64.5%	61.7%	64.7%	64.0%	63.3%	64.7%	62.2%	64.4%	64.5%
31	32	38	50	38	41	56	49	79	69	87	81	80
5.0%	4.7%	5.4%	6.3%	4.3%	4.9%	5.9%	4.8%	7.1%	5.7%	7.0%	6.5%	5.9%
458	489	527	573	656	630	706	739	803	897	857	865	891
74.0%	72.2%	75.4%	72.7%	74.5%	75.0%	74.0%	71.7%	72.2%	73.7%	69.3%	69.4%	66.0%
32	30	33	38	29	34	58	48	63	91	103	87	78
5.2%	4.4%	4.7%	4.8%	3.3%	4.0%	6.1%	4.7%	5.7%	7.5%	8.3%	7.0%	5.8%
85	93	84	108	118	145	161	213	202	214	235	253	247
13.7%	13.7%	12.0%	13.7%	13.4%	17.3%	16.9%	20.7%	18.2%	17.6%	19.0%	20.3%	18.3%
89	109	109	133	116	165	141	192	185	226	236	238	223
14.4%	16.1%	15.6%	16.9%	13.2%	19.6%	14.8%	18.6%	16.6%	18.6%	19.1%	19.1%	16.5%
8.83	8.91	9.00	9.00	9.08	9.59	9.17	9.92	9.63	9.50	9.91	9.79	10.00
35.50	35.96	35.92	36.42	36.75	37.17	37.83	37.75	38.42	37.79	38.08	38.46	38.42

TABLE G-4 Characteristics of the Science and Engineering Workforce in the Basic Biomedical Sciences

	1975	1977	1979	1981	1983	1985	1987	1989	1991	1993	1995	1997
Total	40639	44727	49827	54660	58118	63194	67341	72142	74405	79497	82983	92955
Men	34110	37141	41166	44350	46429	49956	52565	55318	55712	58424	59925	65716
Women	6529	7586	8661	10310	11689	13238	14776	16824	18693	21030	23095	27239
Minorities[a]	1076	1171	1286	1592	1561	1862	1950	2251	2805	3048	3410	3943
Citizens	38187	41756	46158	51499	55337	60153	64015	68451	70501	74398	76570	84887
Permanent residents	1118	1340	1807	2291	2192	2359	2646	2807	2709	3653	5091	4922
Temporary residents	796	1080	1669	503	331	473	581	884	997	1431	1322	1466
Tenured faculty	13376	14345	15636	17836	18884	20114	19157	19755	17106	19151	19487	20326
Tenure track, not tenured	8854	9170	5952	6446	5673	6644	6149	5872	7556	7683	8259	8974
Total academics	27219	29889	33188	36165	36797	39307	41027	43572	40581	45247	48568	53026
Tenured or tenure-track faculty	22230	23515	21588	24282	24557	26758	25306	25627	24662	26834	27746	29300
Nontenure-track faculty	668	1057	4476	3586	3953	3696	5974	6235	4010	5386	5713	6822
Academic postdoctorates	2615	3507	4358	4722	4405	4450	4784	5993	4819	6401	7693	9620
Other academics	1706	1810	3092	3575	3882	4403	4963	5717	7090	6626	7427	7296
Total industry[b]	5326	5583	6313	7951	9635	11967	13588	15582	18513	19950	19434	22204
Industry professionals	5273	5543	6286	7881	9589	11841	13366	15376	18309	19579	18903	21643
Industry postdoctorates	53	40	27	70	46	126	222	206	204	371	531	561
Total government	4030	4250	4776	4831	5287	5399	6254	6290	6589	7200	7185	8649
Government professionals	3785	3914	4449	4545	4843	5026	5725	5776	6157	6154	6074	7212
Government postdoctorates	245	336	327	286	444	373	529	514	432	1046	1111	1437
Other sectors of employment	3055	3436	4103	4303	4657	5043	4847	5034	5984	4072	3790	5602

[a] African Americans, Hispanics, and Native Americans; tabulations include U.S. citizens and permanent residents only.
[b] Including those who are self-employed.

SOURCE: Data are from the Survey of Doctorate Recipients.

TABLE G-5 Characteristics of the Science and Engineering Workforce in the Behavioral and Social Sciences

	1975	1977	1979	1981	1983	1985	1987	1989	1991	1993	1995	1997
Total	25802	29155	33010	36662	41038	43862	45295	48844	48154	51307	52324	57843
Men	20501	22569	25033	27006	29315	30171	30392	31896	30151	31485	30959	33605
Women	5301	6586	7977	9656	11723	13691	14903	16948	18003	19849	21365	24238
Minorities[a]	642	843	1049	1444	1774	1846	1980	2274	2760	3042	3278	4015
Citizens	25170	28556	31993	35664	39918	42559	44107	47449	46565	49746	50745	55822
Permanent residents	340	322	569	795	856	1066	1113	1149	1338	1353	1388	1732
Temporary residents	165	127	332	123	182	135	50	218	160	178	178	289
Tenured faculty	10038	11285	12901	14700	16960	17113	15968	17053	15291	17183	18121	19492
Tenure track, not tenured	6803	6729	4506	4538	4169	4759	4041	4359	4597	4974	4790	4879
Total academics	18668	20132	22543	25025	26896	28472	28187	29841	26475	29901	31764	34850
Tenured or tenure-track faculty	16841	18014	17407	19238	21129	21872	20009	21412	19888	22157	22911	24371
Nontenure-track faculty	690	710	2719	2290	2306	2606	3819	3643	2204	2410	2797	3168
Academic postdoctorates	435	543	806	760	702	713	579	745	412	469	967	1177
Other academics	702	865	2119	2737	2759	3281	3780	4041	3971	4865	5089	6134
Total industry[b]	2111	2777	3487	4643	6625	7345	8032	8843	10696	10896	10484	11779
Industry professionals	2111	2773	3487	4643	6622	7328	8029	8838	10696	10878	10421	11650
Industry postdoctorates	0	4	0	0	3	17	3	5	0	18	63	129
Total government	1793	2394	2654	2831	3058	3182	3858	3732	3900	4874	4993	5192
Government professionals	1778	2353	2605	2781	3013	3163	3816	3732	3816	4748	4854	5071
Government postdoctorates	15	41	49	50	45	19	42	0	84	126	139	121
Other sectors of employment	2662	2788	3116	3181	3200	3740	3876	4787	4631	3201	3138	3820

[a] African Americans, Hispanics, and Native Americans; tabulations include U.S. citizens and permanent residents only.
[b] Including those who are self-employed.

SOURCE: Data are from the Survey of Doctorate Recipients.

TABLE G-6 Characteristics of the Science and Engineering Workforce in the Clinical Sciences

	1975	1977	1979	1981	1983	1985	1987	1989	1991	1993	1995	1997
Total	3515	3815	4615	5390	6119	7340	7835	9154	9479	11143	12431	14618
Men	3028	3161	3709	4211	4560	5117	5139	5603	5416	5752	5826	6918
Women	487	654	906	1179	1559	2223	2696	3551	4063	5352	6605	7700
Minorities[a]	134	146	186	201	260	281	348	500	626	762	946	1139
U.S. citizens	3276	3515	4207	4977	5766	6917	7334	8647	8929	10483	11669	13635
Permanent residents	125	170	264	362	336	340	446	435	471	467	693	775
Temporary residents	83	91	148	44	8	79	55	72	65	184	69	208
Tenured faculty	931	1031	1271	1424	1516	1968	1960	2191	1890	2331	2770	3081
Tenure track, not tenured	684	743	565	780	921	1002	931	1337	1426	1749	1988	1878
Total academics	1856	2064	2564	2963	3225	3938	4164	4959	4706	5753	6684	7609
Tenured or tenure-track faculty	1615	1774	1836	2204	2437	2970	2891	3528	3316	4080	4758	4959
Nontenure-track faculty	56	78	423	438	485	443	784	843	761	944	947	1366
Academic postdoctorates	107	108	105	139	100	177	90	152	116	140	342	416
Other academics	78	104	231	182	203	348	399	436	513	589	637	868
Total industry[b]	739	733	992	1259	1493	1798	1954	2310	2568	2867	2940	3617
Industry professionals	739	733	992	1259	1485	1793	1940	2307	2564	2862	2923	3568
Industry postdoctorates	0	0	0	0	8	5	14	3	4	5	17	49
Total government	500	470	457	562	619	703	753	918	1080	1207	1410	1514
Government professionals	491	462	446	527	585	689	745	916	1064	1141	1309	1467
Government postdoctorates	9	8	11	35	34	14	8	2	16	66	101	47
Other sectors of employment	380	455	436	501	645	749	760	778	847	828	962	1329

[a]African Americans, Hispanics, and Native Americans; tabulations include U.S. citizens and permanent residents only.
[b]Including those who are self-employed.

SOURCE: Data are from the Survey of Doctorate Recipients.

TABLE G-7 Primary Form of Financial Support for Graduate Students in the Basic Biomedical Sciences

Mechanisms of Support	1975	1977	1979	1981	1983	1985	1987	1989	1991	1993	1995	1997
NIH and other DHHS traineeships and fellowships	5068	4281	4363	3678	3478	3400	3502	3486	3896	4001	4138	3941
NIH and other DHHS research assistantships	1832	2227	2804	3092	3159	3608	4562	5918	6483	7174	7461	7436
Other federal support	1897	2322	2509	2579	2407	2581	2651	2854	3087	3690	3800	3816
Institutional teaching assistantships	7530	7703	8076	8160	8200	8150	7547	7736	7685	7866	8005	7861
Other institutional support	4195	5865	5304	5811	6061	6816	8212	8991	10006	10435	10946	10819

SOURCE: Data are from the Survey of Graduate Students and Postdoctorates in Science and Engineering.

TABLE G-8 Primary Source of Financial Support for Graduate Students in the Behavioral and Social Sciences

Mechanisms of Support	1975	1977	1979	1981	1983	1985	1987	1989	1991	1993	1995	1997
NIH and other DHHS traineeships and fellowships	3666	3139	2664	1381	665	625	523	457	575	539	540	563
NIH and other DHHS research assistantships	867	916	946	668	590	681	744	1015	1139	1242	1179	1236
Other federal support	2146	2546	1842	2744	2150	2045	2069	2129	2310	2458	2532	2560
Institutional teaching assistantships	7186	7215	7268	7705	7686	7852	8112	8579	8795	9581	9724	9801
Other institutional support	5311	5948	5724	6663	6827	7423	7926	8908	9815	10411	10249	10828

SOURCE: Data are from the Survey of Graduate Students and Postdoctorates in Science and Engineering.